MW01256722

ALSO BY RAYMOND ANTROBUS

Poetry

The Perseverance

All the Names Given

Signs, Music

Picture Books

Can Bears Ski?

Terrible Horses

The Quiet Ear

The Quiet Ear

An Investigation of Missing Sound

A MEMOIR

Raymond Antrobus

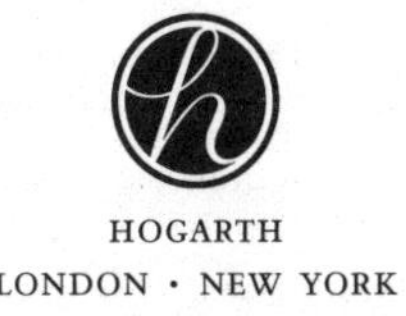

HOGARTH
LONDON · NEW YORK

Hogarth
An imprint of Random House
A division of Penguin Random House LLC
1745 Broadway, New York, NY 10019
randomhousebooks.com
penguinrandomhouse.com

Hardback ISBN 978-0-593-73210-6
Ebook ISBN 978-0-593-73211-3

Printed in the United States of America on acid-free paper

2 4 6 8 9 7 5 3 1

1st Printing

FIRST EDITION

The authorized representative in the EU for product safety and compliance is Penguin Random House Ireland, Morrison Chambers, 32 Nassau Street, Dublin D02 YH68, Ireland, https://eu-contact.penguin.ie.

To my family,
blood and found

Half-heard and half-created.

—William Wordsworth

We have more senses than we have words for,
so perhaps we ought to revel in that if we are
to truly live our lives in the light.

CONTENTS

AUTHOR'S NOTE

Note on D/deaf

The terms Deaf and deaf are interchanged throughout this text. The big "D" Deaf represents culturally Deaf signing people who embrace Deaf identity and culture. The small "d" represents deafened people who use speech. This is a general law, coded within Deaf culture worldwide.

Note on B/black

The terms Black and black are interchanged throughout this text. The big "B" Black often represents the Black (North American) culture and context, which positions Blackness as a primary identity and culture. The small "b" black is used to refer to wider diasporic B/black identities, in which not all black-identifying people subscribe to capitalizing the *B*, including in Africa, the Caribbean, Asia, and Europe. This is my own stylistic choice for this particular text; there is no general law.

The Quiet Ear

Introduction

In 2019, at a turn in my life, when I had just been announced as the winner of an award for my first poetry collection, I was ushered into a back room and took a call from a BBC journalist. I put the phone on loudspeaker and angled it toward the microphone on my hearing aids.

"Congratulations, Mr. Antrobus!" came the low-pitched BBC voice. I could make out around 60 percent of what was said, then I filled the rest in myself. This is how most spoken conversations work for me: I gather up the words I can hear and guess at the missing sounds. The same is true for any conversation, but because of that steady, radio-trained baritone voice, and because I could guess the line of questioning, I thought I could—to my relief—navigate that exchange efficiently.

The very first question felt like an indictment. "It's my understanding that you're deaf, so how are you able to talk to me now?" Why ask this straightaway and live on air? I explained as best I could, but the journalist sounded almost disappointed by how clearly I spoke. I wasn't the kind of deaf person that he expected to speak to.

For many, a deaf person is only one thing: someone profoundly deaf who cannot hear anything even with hearing aids. Someone who can only sign and perhaps lip-read. In reality, deaf identity exists on a continuum; it always has and it always will. At no point in history was there a singular universal deaf experience.

There are people who miss different ranges of sound within different intensities and start to miss them at different times in their lives. In addition, D/deaf identity comes with its own histories, languages, and sensibilities, as much as any culture and subculture. There are as many regional accents and slang in sign language as there are in spoken language, often with wildly different signs that hold the same meaning.

So where do I fit on this continuum? How deaf am I? I was born with high-frequency deafness, meaning that without hearing aids I am unable to hear high-pitched sounds, like doorbells ringing, kettles whistling, or birds singing. At the same time, I have moderate deafness in low-frequency, deeper-pitched sounds. So, in any sentence, even one delivered by a BBC journalist, I will miss parts of words and some words altogether. For example, I often hear the word "suspicious" as "spacious," one syllable completely swallowed, missing, disappeared, even when reading it on the lips.

Capital "D" Deaf people (meaning culturally Deaf people, who sign as a first language and are engaged in deaf history and identity) might classify me as "hard of hearing," and sometimes

I get so tangled up in other people's assumptions, stereotypes, and confusions of deafness that I defiantly call myself "hard of hearing" too. It often doesn't require any follow-up questions. But "hard of hearing" is generally a label for nonsigning, late-deafened people, and it doesn't capture my experience of deafness.

This is all I've ever known, and for a long time I didn't know others around me had a different, fuller experience of sound. When I did, I still could not find a medical template for my deafness that made sense to my experience. "Hearing loss," "hearing impaired," "sensorineural hearing loss" were all labels applied to me by different hearing specialists, but none of them was wholly appropriate to me as someone who was born with my degree of deafness.

I could not begin to explain all this as I struggled in that BBC interview. I felt, though, that I shouldn't have to. Perhaps the best antidote was to get curious, become an investigator of my missing sounds. The idea of curating and examining my relationship with sound felt liberating as a deaf person and a creative thinker. It felt communal, an invitation, a challenge to myself and others to build a cultural lineage, to explore and discover the thinkers and artists who navigated their own missing sound in their own way. They became my co-investigators and the mentors and role models I had missed as a child.

So, what exactly is missing sound? Missing sound is a sound not heard within your range of hearing and, as I explored, as well as finding joy and nourishment in that so-called missingness, I charted losses too. Missing sound can also be interpreted as a misunderstanding, a mismanaged sense of self, a miseducation, a miscellaneous shelf in a mystery library.

Another connotation of "sound" is safety: to arrive somewhere "safe and sound" is to be settled; to be "sound" is to be thorough, well balanced, well adjusted—these are the kinds of qualities most of us seek as humans, no? If sound is missing, it implies something is needed. Whose fault is it that this was not given to me and how do I find it?

If no one is at fault, how do I channel the torment it can bring to be without sound?

I live with the aid of deafness. Like poetry, it has given me an art, a history, a culture, and a tradition to live through. This book charts that art in the hopes of offering a map, a mirror, a small part of a larger story. This book is not a polemic, not an argument for sign language; nor is it against speech therapy or cochlear implants. It is an investigation: an attempt to capture an honest account of how my experience of deafness and betweenness has formed me, from boyhood to parenthood, and how it's impacted my own relationship to language—spoken, written, and signed.

1

The Frequencies Are Yours

Let me go back then, to the sounds of my birth.

If I close my eyes, the sounds of my birth come from a million places at once. Wind in the trees by the beeping traffic on the main road, the shrilling bike bells under the canal bridges, the bustling markets, trolleys rolling over grazed pavements, the clanging of the market-stall bars, the "pound a bowl, pound a bowl" yelling, road works drilling, digging, engines whirring, shutters clanging, the shovels coming down on the hot tarmac, the pop and crash of the lifted manhole covers, the radios blaring in the cars and the offices and the open living-room windows, the dogs barking, the rivers running, voices on the train carriages and the buses, bars, galleries, benches by the lake, children on the climbing frame and children who have tucked themselves into the huts and the tunnels on the adventure playgrounds.

They come from the families standing out in the fields clapping as the children's kites flap in the wind, the coo-coo pigeons, the chirp-chirp sparrows, the man scattering seeds beneath the Trafalgar Square lions. The trees with their branches and leaves stretching past the windows of the hospital wards and corridors as if saying *now* or *live* or *breathe* or *hear hear hear.*

In 1986 in Homerton Hospital, London, a midwife clicked her fingers next to my newborn ears and gauged my response. It was my first hearing test, and I passed.

There were so many sounds that existed that I would not hear until I was fitted with hearing aids at the age of seven. Until then, I existed in my own kind of noise.

For the first seven years of my life, it was assumed I was just slow or perhaps dyslexic. I would miss vital details in teachers' instructions, which kept getting me into trouble, like being told I could play outside but missing the "come back in five minutes"; then, during the subsequent detention (a harsh punishment but the teachers thought I was deliberately disobedient), being told to write about why "punctuality was important" and composing a wonky-lined misspelled essay on the value of punctuation. I was constantly told that what I was hearing was wrong without understanding why, which meant I couldn't trust myself or the world around me. How does a child make sense of words or the world when they seem slippery and untrustworthy? What new perspectives and sensibilities might open up during this formative period?

No one knew I was deaf until my mother bought a large, exceptionally loud, cream-colored telephone that sat in her living room like a pet. The phone rang and rang, and my mother looked at me, unresponsive to the shrilling.

This is how I was diagnosed as deaf.

At a children's audiology clinic in Hackney called the Donald Winnicott Centre, I sat in a small room with my mother and a serious-looking woman in a white, thickly knitted sweater. I was seven years old. I didn't know who or what Donald Winnicott was but I thought he must be old because that's how the clinic felt: brown and gray carpets in sterilized waiting rooms. My mother sat in the corner of that small, soundproofed room with padded walls. The serious-looking woman sat behind a big cream-colored machine with yellow and green buttons.

"Raymond," my mum said slowly. She spoke to me differently when we were inside this building. Her voice slower, louder. I heard her as she looked at me, her face serious as she handed me a gray remote with one black button on it. "The doctor wants you to press this button when you hear a sound."

I faced the serious doctor; her eyes were on the lights on her machine. Every now and then I heard a creepy sound, like a ghost whistling faintly, so I pressed the black button and the sound disappeared.

After the doctor turned off the machine she only had one expression: a look of concentration, with raised eyebrows and tight forehead, which held permanent suspense. It gave Mum a hard listening face when she looked at her, but it softened every time she turned away to look at me.

Mum and I sat, parked outside the clinic in her red Mini Metro. I knew she had something important to say because she put on both our seatbelts and didn't start the engine. "Raymond, I heard every one of those sounds in that room and I didn't see you press the button." She looked scared, whereas I remember feeling deeply impressed that she could hear things that weren't there. She didn't explain what this meant, but the test had revealed the hidden nuance of my hearing.

Shortly after, I was fitted with my first hearing aids. In a school photo taken at the time, you'll see I'm not wearing hearing aids. I would whip them out whenever my photo was being taken, mainly out of shame. In my childhood journals, I wrote that "hearing aids don't suit me" because they highlighted my vulnerability and made me feel ugly, incapable, and "disabled."

It was around this time that I began discovering my missing sounds: anything high-pitched—whistles, birds, kettles, alarms; "sh, ch, ba, th" sounds in speech—the slow vibrating wavelengths that were meant to be picked up by small hair cells in my inner ear; all of them missing.

My parents had to navigate this world of deafness for me. They were both hearing, as were all the medical professionals I met, and everyone emphasized my deafness as a "loss," something that would require effort to manage in the hearing world. I would sit in audiology clinics or at the front of classrooms or even around tables in special educational needs (SEN) units and I would only be assessed and understood as someone struggling to hear.

Once, while I was being dropped off at school, the mother of one of my school friends told me my mother was overreacting by giving me hearing aids because I didn't seem deaf enough. But my parents knew. They saw how loud I had to turn up the television, how often there were gaps in my understanding, and how I didn't answer the door or the phone.

In 2021, within an hour of my son's birth he was given a hearing test. His mother and I watched the doctors set up the machine as he lay wrapped in blankets, our eyes wide and unblinking as wires were attached to his ears. The machine whirred and beeped; his head wobbled. The doctor peered at the graph, muttered "Good," and rushed away, the machine disappearing down the corridor.

I was anxious the doctors might have got it wrong. No one showed me my son's audiogram; I had to take the doctor's "good" word for it. But "good" so often fails to pick up nuances. "Good" failed me in this context. "Good." That vague but affirming word, the word God used when looking over "all He had made."

I began to wonder how my hearing son's experience would differ from mine, and how we might understand or misunderstand each other. For over ten years I'd worked as a freelance poetry teacher, mainly in secondary schools. As a teacher I appreciated the need to scaffold ideas and model behavior; I wondered how I would do this for my son, and I wondered how I ever did it for myself.

Since my son's birth, the African proverb "It takes a village to raise a child" keeps running through my mind. I take stock of my community, parents, deaf people, writers, artists—and I turn to Granville Redmond.

Born in the second half of the nineteenth century, Redmond was a Deaf painter, actor, and mime artist. Art critics at the time had different things to say about Redmond's deafness and how elements of his identity were expressed in his paintings. They described his scenes as "muted" and "silent." Some thought the loud color of his paintings was a result of his deafness, while others thought the quieter nocturnal paintings and tonalist paintings represented what Redmond called his "solitude and silence." Much depended on who was writing about Redmond and what they projected onto him. Redmond, however, didn't resist this kind of categorizing. He suggested that he had developed his style of landscape painting because he had experienced "the loss of other senses."

Redmond's full name was Granville Richard Seymour Redmond, known to his family simply as Seymour, the same name as my father.

On a virtual tour of Redmond's 2020 exhibition (The Eloquent Palette), a painting appears of the exact scene I had seen in many of my dreams since becoming a father. It's called *Sunset over Lake* and is part of a series of nocturnal paintings Redmond created in the early 1900s.

Redmond's paintings became known for their quiet scenes that cry out in almost psychedelic color, and yet there's always something gentle about his touch despite the dramatic tones, particularly in his coastal landscapes of California. Violet, orange, yellow flowers are scattered in the foreground of many of his paintings; rocks and patches of earth between all the wild grass and plant life hinting at paths grown over. You can spend so much time taking in the vibrancy of the flowers alone (especially the golden poppies) that it takes a while to notice how often there is water, a shore, distant hills, and a bright sky keeping the same company, even taking up more of the canvas. On a Redmond canvas, beauty is as much the rock in the grit as the torn pieces of clouds in the sky. Every object in his landscape is rendered with his radiant spirit.

People rarely show up in Redmond's paintings, but when

they do they're seen from a distance, faces muted in contrast to the landscape. Their main purpose seems to be to offer a sense of scale for the trees, hills, flowers, sky, shore, landscape, so you can feel shrunk by it, a threshold into something larger. With a brush in his hand, he brightened, and was not afraid to be guided by his passions.

"Something puzzles me about Redmond's pictures," said his friend Charlie Chaplin in 1925, who purchased a number of Redmond's works and hung them on the walls of his mansion. "There's such a wonderful joyousness about them all. Look at the gladness in that sky, the riot of color on those flowers. Sometimes I think that the silence in which he lives has developed in him some sense, some great capacity for happiness in which we others are lacking." I wonder what the most visibly recognizable silent-film actor of all time knew about *living* in silence.

Redmond's deafness was a result of contracting scarlet fever as a toddler. The same disease afflicted Redmond's son at the same age. At this time Redmond was painting storms. In *Coastal Storm* (1905) a single tree is blown viciously, its leaves torn away in the turbulence, and the huge, dark black-gray sky seems to be just beginning; long needle-like streaks of rain pour down diagonally to illustrate the force and drama of the wind. In the center of the picture is a thin footpath, barely visible, cutting through the grass leading toward a distant opening of bright shore, blue sea. I keep looking at that turbulent tree, imagining Redmond himself, the dark sky spread before him, and he's standing before it, brush in hand.

Does this say something about the lines of imagined, felt, and lived trauma? Was Seymour, sorry, Granville projecting his anxious existential feelings? Did his son get swept away in it, even after surviving the illness? How much of fatherhood is simply what we make of it? How much of fatherhood is simply weathering a storm?

My son is in my arms; it's June, his first summer on Earth, and we are in swimming costumes and walking into the warm Schlachtensee lake in Berlin. Families lay towels and picnic blankets under the trees in the small bays that are the most generously shady. It's my first time swimming with my son. His shoulders are tense and he clings to my chest, digging his nails into my arms; he peers down at the dark water, which is up to my waist, and I wade forward slowly, getting deeper.

"Hello, lake, hello, water," I say, demystifying the scene. I name each witness of this moment; my son looks at me, a mix of confusion and voracious curiosity. "Da-da?" he says, then he looks at the lake, "Da-da?," then the surrounding trees and the glowing sun, "Da-da?"

I heave into the depth where our bodies submerge but our heads bob above the surface, the lake warmed by the sun.

If Redmond painted this scene, it'd be called *Summer Lake;* the sun, high and blazing above the trees, could be a day-moon. My son and I would be muted blotches, our faces featureless, like planets through a telescope, the water a green-black varnished surface, dark and shining. Each tree around the lake would be given its detail: wide arms, curling twigs and branches, different complexions on the bark, and a generous casting of shadows on the water; the water wouldn't offer either my son or me our reflections.

Or maybe Redmond would choose to paint the moment my son and I submerged beneath the water, completely disappearing from my medium of words and into his quieter color. He'd dabble the ripples to hint at a presence: We could be fish gawping close to the surface, diving ducks, sinking stones, or small rippling vibrations. If my son saw the painting, he'd probably point at that spot, and say:

Da-da?

According to Nicholas Mirzoeff's book *Silent Poetry,* in Roman mythology, Saturn was thought to be the inventor of speech. The most famous of deaf painters, Francisco Goya, created his canonical "Black Paintings"—including *Saturn Devouring His Son* (1823)—as a deaf man. Spanish Sign Language became his primary mode of communication. Perhaps the Saturn figure consuming his child on Goya's canvas represents an exorcism of his hearing self and the violent tearing of his connection to the hearing world?

My deafness means that I require tools and methods to help me navigate the hearing world. Hearing aid technology has come a long way in the thirty years since I began wearing them. I can lip-read well thanks to my NHS speech therapist, who spent hours facing me with her mouth open, instructing me where to place a finger on my throat so I could feel the vibration of sounds I couldn't hear, sounding out the words and the position of my teeth, tongue, and lips. Lip-reading and speech therapy are controversial in deaf education. They have been used to force profoundly deaf people to use speech rather than sign language, which was believed to delay a deaf person's literacy skills and assimilation into mainstream hearing society. These puritanical educators founded what is called "oralism"—a teaching method used to educate deaf students through speech and lip-reading rather than sign language—a practice popularized by many nineteenth-century proponents and advocates of the time, most notably the Scottish-born inventor of the telephone (1876), Alexander Graham Bell.

Since English is my first language, if I sign I mostly use SSE (Sign Supported English) to communicate with the D/deaf, rather than traditional BSL (British Sign Language). I was taught BSL at school but I refused to use it out of self-consciousness. I was embarrassed to be seen signing it in front of hearing kids or anyone outside of the deaf school. My sign style was improvised, nontraditional, and represented how loosely and reluctantly integrated I was in the deaf world.

For me, lip-reading worked for my level of deafness but I was able to incorporate what I learned from hearing speech therapists and Deaf BSL teachers to form my own hybrid D/deaf identity. I make a convincing listening face, even if I'm only half understanding a conversation. I've learned to accept what I receive; it sometimes makes me appear goofy, aloof, or eccentric to hearing people, but I've worked through years of self-consciousness to earn an ease with this. People have to understand that they are talking to a deaf person, and quite often they forget because of how well I mask it, how "clear my speech is," how powerful my hearing technology is, and how seamlessly I pick up the etiquettes of hearing people.

The sound I had as a child is a world away from the sound I access now with high-powered digital technology. But what have I lost in the amplification? Am I losing my deaf sense, my "eye music," a term coined by Wordsworth that deaf poet David Wright used to frame his deaf poetic sensibility—the mode that gifted Granville Redmond his "eloquent palette" and Francisco Goya his canonical "Black Paintings"?

Have I dulled my ability to hyper-tune in to the visual? If our real identity lies in "inner speech," as psychologist Lev Semyonovich Vygotsky states, have I lost that? My real identity? Has my so-called improved access to sound taken away my natural deaf disposition?

I decided to experiment by not wearing hearing aids for a week, to return to a duller sound where speech has more holes. Birdsong, alarms, buzzers, kettles—all higher frequencies would disappear from my life again and I would be met without the inventions and interventions of hearing technology that I have come to rely on.

My first morning hearing aid–less, my son is eating a bowl of porridge at the table. He raises his spoon and says something. I stare at his lips; I can't make it out.

"Ra-ra?"

I stare at him blankly. His eyes get wider.

"Ra-ra!?"

He kicks his feet under the table and throws his spoon on the floor.

I go through the signs that we've been practicing. "Milk?" "Food?" "Open?"

His mother walks into the room. "I think he's asking for water?"

I sign "water." He doesn't repeat it; he's too flustered. He raises his arms.

"Up, up!"

He wants his mother to lift him out of our misunderstanding.

His mother and I notice how quickly frustrated our son gets

when he isn't understood. This is a trait I see in myself, a panicky sensitivity to misunderstandings, maybe because of being raised in a (nonculturally Deaf) hearing family. Seeing it in my son makes me wonder again about what is "natural" to me and to our family.

With his hands, my son is communicating his first words. Language is beginning. His finger-pointing is *you? this? that?*—a straightened question mark.

His spoken language is forming too, like a mushy ball of clay; his "good" hearing and his natural determined focus have put his verbal language acquisition on track. Even his resting face is thoughtful; his sounds often end with question marks: *Da-da? Ma-ma? Na-na?*

He points at me with his finger, a strikingly deliberate point, a "God on the creation of Adam on the Sistine Chapel ceiling" kind of point. I, like Adam in the painting, reach toward him to point back, to mimic his gesture. There is something new and commanding about it.

He's curious about people, stares at strangers on park benches and at bus stops, waves at them, but he loves dogs and birds the most, gets particularly animated in his stroller when he sees them; he gazes, points, wants to get closer. He is also drawn to trees and plants: the wider the leaves, the more excited he is to greet them; he strokes them with the same careful, curious touch that he gave to a puppy that once wandered up to him while he sat on the grass in the park.

Da-da?

My son is not deaf. His development has already surpassed mine at his age. Where I was slow to walk and talk, he can stand up and step forward without stumbling. I'm well aware now, as a new parent, of how development ought to look, its timeline, its list of milestones. It sends me back to my own.

My language and communication sensibilities took years to nurture, I'm not me without this experience. It also took me years to reframe my deafness as a gain rather than a loss. The phrase "Deaf gain" was coined by British performing artist Arron Williamson in 2005, after noting his confusion with the term "hearing loss." Williamson asked the question, "Why hearing loss and not gaining deafness?"

Deaf gain was something I had to come to on my own too, well away from schools and medical institutions, and now I start to wonder if there is anything my son might be losing out on by being hearing, by meeting all those expected timelines and milestones. My experience of having lived between the deaf and hearing worlds has offered me much hard-won strength and insight, a particular lens to see the world through.

How could I pass this on? How might I be able to relate to my hearing child? How might my son feel safe around me as a deaf man? Where are the stories and lives that could help me explain?

2

Livin' in Hackney, No One Can Jack Me . . .

Hackney in the 1980s and '90s was one of the most impoverished places in London, yet artists flocked to it for the cheap rent and warehouses. My mother was one of them. She and her twin brother were the youngest of four children of Christian ministers who were pacifists during the Second World War. She was raised in Hemel Hempstead and lived in different parts of Hertfordshire depending on where her father, J.K. Antrobus, was stationed. He went by a few names: Jesse, Keith, Mister or Minister Antrobus, but he preferred to be called J.K. He was a sharply dressed man, with a narrow head, square jawline, slightly wavy hair. Grandma said he always wore gray jackets and trimmed his mustache. I remember her clasping her hands, leaning back in her chair, a black-and-white photo of J.K. beside her, grinning out of the frame, his wavy hair, his neat old-timey handsomeness, and exclaiming, "Kissing a man without a mustache is like eating a boiled egg without salt."

Grandfather J.K. Antrobus died nine months before I was born and I have often wondered what he, as a Christian minister, would have made of my deafness. Christianity often relies on the idea of people with disabilities needing miracle cures rather than community and an integrated sense of acceptance and empowerment. There were no known deaf people in our family before me, so how would J.K. have navigated a deaf grandchild?

He once gave a sermon reflecting on Saint Bernadette, the patron of the sick. Bernadette Soubirous was fourteen in 1858 when she had a series of visions of the Virgin Mary, leading to the founding of the shrine of Lourdes.

Many pilgrims have traditionally visited Lourdes seeking a cure for ailments including deafness. Marie Bigot was the most recent confirmed miracle: She had lost her sight and hearing in 1952, which were restored while she was taking part in a "procession of the blessed Sacrament" after three visits to Lourdes.

In the first paragraph of his sermon, J.K. stops short of calling Bigot's healing a miracle, instead referring to it as a "possible supernatural occurrence," but as the lesson concludes he quotes John 20:28: "So, you believe because you've seen with your own eyes. Even better blessings are in store for those who believe without seeing."

This is a frequent mode of J.K.'s sermons, speculative, expansive, considerate of other cultures, faiths, and languages, but, in his closing, he limits his points to platitudes. He seemed both intellectually expanded and narrowed by his faith.

Neither J.K. nor my grandmother Barbara Antrobus went to traditional university: She was educated in what she called "a prim and proper, local, little private school run by a woman called Miss Oliver" until she was sixteen years old. Private education wasn't the extreme cost it is now; many lower-middle-class families could afford it.

As teenagers, Barbara and J.K. met at Crowstone Congregational Church in Southend-on-Sea, a church known for what some called "radical ideas" like pacifism, gender and racial equality, and equity, things that Quakers and Unitarians also see as true Christian values.

J.K. left secondary education at fourteen and worked at a builders yard, selling cement, bricks, hammers, and nails. Meanwhile, Barbara worked in London for an insurance company, commuting daily from Southend, where she was raised. She had wished to be a children's nurse but for reasons unknown, her grandfather refused to support it. Barbara supported J.K. financially when he left the builders yard and went to study at the Theological College at Haverstock Hill in London, where, in his early twenties, he trained to be a Congregational minister.

Once J.K. became a minister, both the same age, they married at twenty-eight and went on to have four children. After marriage, Barbara quit her insurance post and co-ran the church, describing her new job as "a minister's wife." As well as their own children (Felicity, Rosemary, Christopher, and Michael), J.K. and Barbara fostered a child, Ruby, from a children's home in Bolton. Felicity was working there as a young nurse and simply brought three-year-old Ruby home. J.K. and Barbara stepped in to offer stability to a child in a turbulent care system.

They were never rich: The church owned the houses they lived in and their money came from Christian charity funds and government benefits.

I have a memory of standing in the pews beside my grandmother and sister on a Sunday morning among the congregation. The deep sound of the organ pressed through the echoey church as sunlight illuminated the stained glass above us. Our booklets open with words to the hymns in black text, we began singing and to me it was noise I couldn't decipher. I looked at the text completely flabbergasted that the noise I was hearing had words. It might as well have been a chorus of people babbling *la-la-la-la-la-laaaaa.*

Afterward, the priest, a slim, white-haired, spectacled man, stood at the open doors, shaking hands with the congregation as they filed out. He turned to me, asked:

"Did you enjoy the hymns?"

But I thought he'd said "hums."

"Yes," I said, "I enjoyed the hums."

My mother, Rosemary, was born in 1948, sister to her twin brother, Christopher. One of her earliest memories is being in the twin pram Barbara pushed along the high street as people poked their faces in, cooing, pinching her cheeks. Another is looking out the window at the large house across the street, envying the size and scale, daydreaming of life inside the walls until she learned that it was in fact an orphanage.

When my mother was three, she remembers her mother staring at the crackling fire in the fireplace, lost, not there. She learned that terror is quiet. Barbara had been infected with dysentery, a disease common in England in the late 1940s.

She had four young children when she succumbed to the illness; she lost herself, her family lost her. Barbara was committed to an asylum for three months while J.K. and Mrs. Smith, a woman from his congregation, stepped in to care for the children.

The first house my mother grew up in still stands behind the Alexandra Road Congregational Church in Hertfordshire. Coincidentally, as I write this, I live fairly near this church. I can walk a few miles through the field beside my rented house and be within sightlines from the highest point of the local hills.

Viewed from the street outside, it's a wide-windowed, four-bedroom autumn-brown brick house; a chestnut tree at the back gently wafts in the wind, flat gray pavement and smooth black tarmac road at the front, a symmetrical wooden fence surrounding the house like straightened teeth. It is a comfortable middle-class aesthetic designed to blend in with the street, at odds with the rationing and class struggle of the times. My mother, as the younger-twin sister, sensed this polite effort to convey basic goodness and manners at all times, to never let your problems inconvenience others, to never raise your head above expectation, to project emotional and financial stability. The worst thing she could become, she was told, was "common." It suffocated her.

J.K.'s sermons often evoked the power of image, the need for values to be modeled. The minister's family were self-conscious pillars of their community, but it came at a cost to their children, who couldn't feel important unless they too were involved in outwardly worthy causes. My mother's twin brother became a police officer, her older sister an NHS nurse. Her eldest brother became one of the earliest computer studies students at Salford University and he would never shake his feeling of inferiority, of his work failing to give him a sense of worth and spiritual reward.

A lone rebel among her siblings, my mother left home at eighteen. She thrived academically and pursued higher education, studying English literature at Lancaster University. She found the work too rigid and standardized, the radical writers she admired left off the curriculum; although she took to Bertrand Russell, Kenneth Patchen, and Malcolm Lowry, they weren't enough to sustain her ideological rebelliousness. Her favorite writer was the Marxist-humanist, pan-Africanist philosopher Frantz Fanon, a name unfamiliar to her professors.

She dropped out at the end of her last year, deliberately flunked her exams and became a circus clown, designing inflatable giants with her partner, the English performance artist and clown Jules Baker. They toured the UK, putting on shows and exhibitions while squatting in houses and flats, before settling in east London.

My mother moved through life on instinct: no major plan, just enough self-awareness to know what skills of hers would get her by. They squatted in a house in Hackney, then bought it. Jules started taking on too much work for my mother to keep up, so she dropped the clowning and became an antiques dealer, working down Camden Passage, a narrow pedestrian back street in an aspirational part of north London, full of enterprising people building independent businesses such as antiques shop owners and market traders.

Now she had a house and financial independence, but her relationship with Jules was strained; he had become more reclusive, burying himself in work, and when she demanded his attention, he was occasionally violent. What was meant to be a romantic holiday to the Red Sea turned abusive and my mother wanted to break off the relationship and return to Hackney.

There's a picture of my mother at this time, her long, straight dark brown hair, her eyes pale blue, smooth legs bared and crossed. She's staring out of the shot, away from the camera, as if the picture was taken candidly; there's almost a blur in the photo, a determination in her posture, as if even in this moment of rest, she knows she'll have to move, there's always so much to be done.

In 1978, the night my father met my mother, he was standing behind the turntables at some squatters' party in Dalston. The shutters on all the windows were closed, beams from the streetlights seeped through the gaps, and my father's fingers dropped the needle on Sam Cooke.

My mother looked up over the dark sea of bopping heads; my father glanced out, caught her eye.

Later, my father passed the music to someone else and went to a room upstairs, where a small crowd of people had gathered, and there he noticed my mother, moved toward her. He was six feet tall, hair trimmed short; my mother stood at five-foot-two.

"You fascinate me," he said to her, leaning in.

"Oh." She looked him up and down. The first thing she noticed was his trousers. They were dark gray suit trousers. Every other man was wearing jeans. She tried not to laugh.

"I'm Seymour," he said, pointing at his eyes, "the more I see the more I see," and my mother burst into charmed laughter, stared back at his smile, his smooth, relaxed jaw, his dark blue blazer. They spoke about the Sam Cooke record my father had been playing downstairs; they spoke about the shaking church of the singer's voice, from his gospels to the pop charts. Seymour liked the fact that Cooke had added an "e" to his name "Cook" in 1957, the year he left Jamaica, marking a new path. He implied he'd added an "e" too, *Sey* to *See*. He told my mother he lived on a street that happened to be round the corner from her. "Come see me sometime."

When he returned to the music downstairs, he played Sam Cooke again:

Oh, won't you bring it on home to me . . .

My mother hadn't officially ended it with Jules, but she remembered my father's address and showed up at the house a few days later. He opened the door in a light blue buttoned-up shirt and holding a rolled-up cigarette. He closed the door behind her and their affair began.

My father also had a partner, Peggy, a gentle East End Cockney woman with a round face and long blond hair. It was her house that my father was living in; it was her bed they slept in. For years the affair played out. Neither Jules (my mother stayed a bit longer, despite his abuse) nor Peggy would find out until my mother fell pregnant with my sister in 1982.

My mother was thirty-two at this point and kept her parents at a distance. They weren't a family that talked heart-to-heart; she couldn't speak to them and trust that she would be understood. She sensed how they worried about her, though, and tried to stay out of the orbit of their anxiety. She was forging her own life and identity. She knew their values, their conventions; knew she was at odds with them. She, a rebel, a smoker, drinker, had sex unmarried. J.K.'s policy was that the children had to find their own way. They knew Rosemary wouldn't grow up and just become a housewife, but they hoped she'd be a teacher, social worker, or missionary, though this was never said out loud. There is something English about the way silence can carry any heavy suppressed emotion.

Now, J.K. and Barbara's concern for their daughter was made concrete. She was pregnant by a man who didn't seem stable, and she had recently broken up with Jules. It shocked them.

Jules had said he never wanted children and Peggy wasn't able to. Jules struck my mother in the face; Peggy cried, broke down, yelled. A few months later Jules ended up staying in the same house as my mother, my father absent and nowhere to be seen. Jules said he'd help raise the child, and he was there, not my father, when my sister was born.

My grandmother Barbara first spoke to my father a few weeks after my mother gave birth to my sister, Corrina. He had called the house after hearing from his friend that my mother was seen pushing a pram with a brown little girl with curly hair down Dalston Lane. My grandmother picked up the phone, realized who it was, and spat down the receiver. The only black men my grandmother had met were book-carrying men of the cloth who visited her husband's church wearing thick-rimmed glasses, stood clean-shaven on pulpits, and preached love and reconciliation while quoting Corinthians, Shakespeare, and Desmond Tutu. She did not know how to process a black man who smoked, drank, and abandoned his child. My father didn't like the way my grandmother spoke to him; he yelled back, *Shut yuh rass, woman*. This only made visceral sense to her. She gasped, called him *black devil*! Although my father would swear she called him *nigger.*

My father was born in Patty Hill, in the Hanover parish of Jamaica, in July 1938, to Darcas James and Porter Birch. "Country" or "bush" is how he referred to his birthplace, located deep in the Jamaican hills of overgrown paths that required a cutlass to clear a path through the plants and branches that blocked the way. The second youngest of seven brothers, he was the only child as dark-skinned as his mother. The other brothers had a caramel complexion, he was mahogany. The fact of this contrast led to teasing: Some kids around the hills noted it with suspicion and mockery, and, despite being in a predominantly black country, it, perhaps, gave my father an "ugly duckling" complex. This was projected onto me in many ways: For example, when my father was drunk he called me "white," when he was sober he called me "black."

When he was three his aunt Avis took him from the bush of Patty Hill to Kingston, the capital city, without warning or explanation. Even when my father told me this story as a sixty-year-old man, his face hardened as he remembered himself as the three-year-old who sat on Aunt Avis's balcony, crying, wailing, hoping his burst sound would reach the hills over the island and signal his father to return him.

Aunt Avis's only child had been stillborn, and it's not clear if my father was given to her as a consolation or because she saw academic potential in him and knew he'd benefit from a "city education." Perhaps both, but my father would always interpret this as abandonment, as if he was sent away because of his dark skin. He spoke vividly of it when he was drunk, a wound that wouldn't close.

While living in Kingston he rarely saw his parents. Porter and Darcas stayed working the land in Patty Hill. Porter was a butcher who set his aspirational sights on England, thinking he could run a lucrative business. Darcas was married off at fifteen and had never left Patty Hill. She tended pigs and fetched water from the waterfalls for washing, cooking, cleaning. In the early 1950s, Porter was the first direct relative of my Jamaican family to board a ship for England.

When my father was six or seven, he wore a light brown school uniform with a yellow tie, his hair trimmed short. It turned out he was indeed academically gifted, so money was pooled from Porter and Avis for his education. My father thrived in class, taking particular interest in English. Most of his classmates were from wealthy families, the children of diplomats, politicians, business owners. He learned Wordsworth and Coleridge poems off by heart and would be brought to the front of the class to recite them. But words were also beaten into him: The teachers kept canes on their desks and swung them at the legs and backs of the children who showed slackness.

One of the boys in my father's class was developmentally slow and struggled with the pressure. The teachers beat him so often that the students turned on him too. The teachers spoke the Queen's English; "yard talk" or patois was prohibited. When one boy, let's call him Calvin, misspoke in class, the teacher swung a lick on his legs with each word: "What. You. Say. Boy. Speak. Up." When Calvin was on the playground outside, another boy walked up to him, a sharpened pencil in each hand, and stabbed him in each ear. Calvin fell to the ground, wailing, a trail of blood running from both sides of his face. Calvin never returned to school, leaving all the students stunned and silent. My father brought up this story whenever my deafness was mentioned. This trauma, his only association with what deafness is. Something that makes you disappear.

Meanwhile, he was popular in school; he had a large group of friends and the teachers recognized his intelligence, sharing his positive reports with Aunt Avis, who thanked the Lord for her nephew's big brain.

Now there's disruption, a tear, a break in the smoother path.

When he was ten, a fifteen-year-old girl forced him into a bush on his way back from school, gave him a bottle of beer, and made him strip, then they had sex. This would be the first time he'd drink alcohol, the first time he'd have sex; this was a story he would tell me if he was drunk, reeling off the anecdote, usually smiling, a dead-eyed recollection.

As a teenager, my father sought out music. He went with friends to live music venues in downtown Kingston in the early 1950s as mento made way for rocksteady and reggae—"heartbeat riddims," I remember my father calling them. Now I must stitch this together, mix it in clean, because it must have been around this time he found DJs and sound technicians in the clubs and studied them, learned how to build his own sound system from discarded amps and wires. It must have been at this point that he first collected records and tapes and played them for his friends at house parties or the tourists by the beach bars.

Aunt Avis noticed the change in her nephew, saw the "rudies," the friends who came knocking for him. They called him

"See," but those who saw him fight called him "Bruck," because "lemme tell yuh, man always ready to bruck up tings."

Aunt Avis took a dislike to my father's friends, calling them a bad influence; she noticed his clothes reeking of tobacco, how he left bottles of Red Stripe under his bed, nodded his head to the Rastas as they passed on the street. But by now my father fully rejected Aunt Avis's values and conventions. She attended the Congregational church in Kingston, buttoned up her shirts and blouses, and sang "The Day Thou Gavest, Lord, Is Ended," and for a while my father stood next to her, sulking in the pews. Then he refused to go. She wrote to his father, Porter, who was already working in England, setting up his butcher shop.

When my father finished his studies, he worked briefly on the railways. In September 1957, the famous Kendal, Manchester, train wreck occurred, killing one hundred and eighty-seven people and injuring seven hundred. To this day it is Jamaica's worst railway disaster. My father felt it was fate: He had escaped death by leaving Jamaica just days beforehand. Porter had sent the money for him to board the ship *Irpinia,* bound for England.

The trip took two weeks and the ship docked in Cuba, Italy, and Spain before arriving at the port of Southampton, on the English south coast. My father had two brothers in Wolverhampton, but everyone he asked for directions sent him to Brixton, "London's Cold Little Jamaica." After his detour back from Brixton, he realized the only jobs that would employ him were the cash-in-hand ones as a bike and car mechanic or painter and decorator. He worked around England, even briefly at Porter's butcher shop as it fell into financial troubles. Promises weren't kept, deeds went missing, money was mismanaged, and the shop had to close. Desperate and strapped for cash, Porter and my father would fall out after my father caught him stealing some of his stashed money—as he had no bank account, cash was hidden in old pairs of socks and tucked into suitcases. Porter returned to Patty Hill and my father moved to London from Wolverhampton. He was employed to paint the corridors of a school in Hackney the week he met my mother at the squatters' party, standing behind all the music.

There was one story that my mother, father, and grandmother Barbara all shared and that's the story of my birth. It might be the only story where they all agree on the facts.

I was born four years after my sister. Jules had left and my father was showing promise as a co-parent, decorating the house that Rosemary had shared with Jules, working steadier jobs, helping her at the market, even taking her and Corrina to Jamaica to meet his parents in Patty Hill. When he got back, he hinted that he would set up his own market stall selling records and tapes. It was in this glowing potential of a future that he told my mother that he wanted a second child.

Nine months later, the Jamaican midwife in Homerton Hospital would click her fingers next to my newborn ears and gauge my response.

When she handed me to my mother, my father leaned in and said: "He looks like a Raymond." The name was put to paper. They wrapped me in blankets and took me to my mother's house in Haggerston, Hackney. While she slept in her bedroom upstairs, builders showed up at the house to repair the roof. The builders stamped their boots on the slates. My father and grandmother sat downstairs in the living room opposite the fireplace. My grandmother held me in her arms as a heavy cloud of soot gushed down the chimney and blackened the walls, windows, carpets, everything. My grandmother, coughing, peered down at my face. I was covered in soot, entirely black. My father laughed when he recounted the story: His focus was on the comedy, part Monty Python sketch, part Richard Pryor stand-up routine—a mixed black child in the arms of his white English grandmother becoming nightmarishly blacker. My grandmother told the story with concern and sincerity, as if it was an omen, a fable, something riddled with tricks and twists, the origins of a wound. My mother tells it anxiously, as if the moral of the story is something practical and economic: Don't fix a roof and birth a child at the same time. But all the elements in their accounts are the same; the only difference between the stories is their tone, slant, shade.

3

Anciently English

I sat in Grandma's living room; she gave me a book with a painting of a young white man, soft blue eyes, thin brown hair combed back, staring out of the cover. Above it the title: *The Collected Poems of Thomas Gray*.

"This is an Antrobus ancestor," she said. "His mother was Dorothy Antrobus," a poor woman from the East End. The opening poem, "Elegy Written in a Country Churchyard," is a dense-metered poem full of sound and feeling that praises the working people who "toil the land," which my mum looked at too, leaning over my shoulder, and said, "Yeah, right on, salt of the earth, mate!" Grandma flicked through one of the Antrobus family albums and showed me a picture of her standing in a field of dark soil wearing shiny black leather shoes and a green overcoat. "Here I am in Antrobus village," she said proudly, as if she owned that land. Antrobus village is in Cheshire. The name

Antrobus is derived from the Norman-French *entre-bois,* meaning "between (or within) the woods." It first appeared in the manuscript of the 1086 Domesday Book. I think of this often. When I return to the UK from international travel, I'm often quizzed at the border by people in uniforms crested with British lions, the words "Border Force" sewn into their blue shirts.

"Antrobus? Where's that from?"

"It's an English name."

"Oh, doesn't sound English."

"It's a village in Cheshire," I explain, offering an annoyingly teachable moment. I have a name so anciently English that it has become foreign to itself.

Years later I visited Antrobus village. I was drafting a manuscript titled *Between the Woods,* with a long poem modeled on Gray's "Elegy." I sat in a tearoom beside Antrobus Farm, told the "tea ladies" I was an Antrobus ancestor, and they made calls, said I should walk toward Antrobus Farm and speak to the people there. On the farm, a bearded man wearing boots and holding a shovel emerged from behind a tractor. "Ah, so Edmund is a relative, is it?" Research had shown me that Sir Edmund Antrobus is the richest Antrobus on record, a slaver and owner of multiple plantations in Jamaica, British Guiana, and St. Kitts. I shook my head, avoided the farmer's eyes.*

Later I was directed toward the cemetery, told there were

*This is a line from the poem "Antrobus or Land of Angels" in *All the Names Given.*

Antrobuses buried there. Sure enough, in St. Mark's churchyard, Antrobus, every grave was marked with the Antrobus name. And, yes, I thought of the land that was toiled and the English working people, the child laborers, the chimney sweeps, the butchers, the blacksmiths, the farmers, the working classes, and I thought of the offshore plantations, the overseers, the tobacco and sugar, the boiling houses, the cotton and the cotton mills, all of it turning, churning, burning, all of it inside the blood pumping in my ears.

When I was four or five, as my parents' relationship was falling apart, my grandmother stepped in, took my sister and me to her Hertfordshire house in Ware during school holidays. My grandfather J.K. had died of leukemia a few years back. He had been taken into King's College Hospital in London and never came out. When I was born, caring for us soothed some of my grandmother's grief and it gave us a comfort we did not know at home in Hackney. She lived in a bungalow with a small brown-and-black dachshund called Coco; she sugared our cereal in the morning, made pink mousse for dessert, boiled potatoes, roasted the chicken, microwaved the gravy; there were always biscuits and mini KitKats in tins in the cupboard, ham sandwiches in a box in the fridge; the electric fire glowed beside the television. A portrait of my silver-haired grandfather with an open palm on the Bible smiled from the mantelpiece and sometimes I would see my grandmother talking to it. I could never make out exactly what she was saying but it seemed like small talk, just recounting her day, her trip to the supermarket, who she saw on the way, who was getting married or moving away or had fallen ill, or how the weather wasn't as warm as was forecast on the BBC.

I never sensed sadness. My grandmother's belief in God, that the dead stay with us, cemented her in this life, kept her present with us and therefore with God and her dead. She also spoke to the birds in her garden, would relay a conversation she'd had with a blue tit, sparrow, or magpie—"they had come to say hello"—sometimes delivering messages from her dead friends, affirming that they were at rest and there was sky and sun and wind wherever they were speaking from. None of this was creepy to me and my sister, but cozily calm and predictable. When my sister moved back in with my mother, she began to resent being at home in Hackney. Because she knew a kind of calm, cozy comfort existed elsewhere, she would make it a priority to find other safer places: friends' houses and quiet parks by ponds with fountains and wooden benches where neighborhood cats ran their bodies along Victorian streetlamps.

My grandmother's music seemed to be all hymns; she had a TV in the kitchen that was only on when *Songs of Praise* was broadcast on BBC One. Sometimes I heard her humming while chopping carrots or opening a tin of custard. "All Things Bright and Beautiful."

She never spoke to me about my father; her worry and disapproval remained silently English. She took it on herself to compensate for what she saw as gaps in my care; love was part of her service and she would deliver it without voicing complaint, but it still existed, quietly in her body, and just a mention of my father's name had her sighing and leaving the room.

When I was diagnosed as deaf, my father and sister were surprised and confused by the news. "But the boy hears me," protested my father. "He'll be fine," my sister said with a shrug. "He's not deaf, he's stupid."

I can't remember the exact order of events, if it was that week, or that year, but around this time my sister and I got into a searing, sloppy fight over something I can't recall. I was just another annoying little brother infuriating his big sister. She hit me hard over the head in front of my father, and I screamed because a sudden, loud imaginary car alarm began blaring in my ears. My father struck my sister back on my behalf.

A week later I complained that I could still hear an imaginary car alarm; my father shunned my sister.

"RASSCLAUT! You made de bwoy deaf!"

That accusation lodged in my sister's mind: that my deafness was something she may have caused. "He'll be fine," she protested, her face red and wet with tears and anger. "He'll be fine!"

My grandmother's response to the news of my hearing test, which my mum framed to her as "Raymond's not hearing one hundred percent," was less alarmist. She suggested my mum ask her sister about it as she was a nurse.

My aunt told my mother not to do grommets, an operation where tiny metal or plastic tubes are surgically inserted into the eardrum, allowing more air to pass through it and unblocking any fluid that might've built up, causing a condition called "glue ear." My aunt advised keeping an eye on it and seeing if it got worse.

A few weeks after my initial test at the Donald Winnicott Centre, I found myself sitting again in a small room with my mother and another doctor, also in a knitted sweater. I remember looking out of the large window, daydreaming, as my mother and the audiologist spoke to each other, then I remember the woman turning to me, directing my focus to her face and away from the sunlit window. She slid a curtain of her hair behind her ear, held up a graph; it showed a steep slope of two lines, red and blue. She explained to Mum that the red line that went down was my hearing curve; most people's line goes straight across. She pointed at the space between the lines. They had discovered the sound I was missing.

"Raymond," said the woman with a warm, consoling smile. *We have discovered that you can't hear any of the sounds between this red and blue line—do you see how the shape of this graph is like a ski slope? You have ski slope deafness.*

Everything about this was magical to me. When I was growing up, Hackney was concrete, full of council blocks and cracked pavements, a world away from ski slopes, mountains, or anything scenically adventurous.

When I was back at the clinic the third time, I saw the serious doctor again. She squeezed white gooey dough into her rubber gloves. The dough smelled like my He-Man toy that I once left on a hot radiator overnight. Then the doctor had another tube of paste that she squeezed onto the dough and turned it blue, like a piece of sky, the exact color of the icing on my Thomas the Tank Engine cake on my fourth birthday. (I made a wish but I won't say what it was.)

The doctor put the blue piece of sky into a large syringe and injected it into my ear. It felt cold but also relaxing because it blocked my ears and took all my sound away.

Without sound I became more aware of my body. My shoulders were tense, so I relaxed them. I don't think anything had ever touched the walls in my ear before. It tickled. I liked the feeling.

The serious doctor spoke with my mother while the mold hardened in my ear. I heard nothing but it made me more aware of the room and the movements in it: faces, bodies, the trays on the doctor's desk, the broken blinds and the clear tubes and the machines.

When the serious doctor unblocked my ears, she showed me a blue cast shaped like my ear. *This is a mold of your ear.*

Two weeks later I would be back in that chair with the second knitted-sweater doctor holding a cast of my ear, but this time it was a clear color, like a piece of window. Then she picked up the pinkish micro-machine-looking device on her desk, a hue that she described as "skin-colored"—but it was her color, not mine.

"This is your device."

"My plastic ear?"

"Yes."

"Will I still be deaf like a ski slope?"

"Yes, but these will help."

She pushed the molds into my ear canals and placed the pinkish machines behind the ears. She flicked a switch on the devices. Sound opened a new mouth filled with walkie-talkie static. I sat inside the faraway staticky breathing of the world. I could hear the cars on the street, the engines approaching us then fading away like the world was swallowing them. It felt harsh and treacherous, like a metal world full of stiff, inescapable crushing machines.

"How's that?"

The doctor's smile was fixed, but her voice sounded louder

and more serious, like a robot's. It frightened me. I looked at Mum. She was smiling but it looked forced because I could tell from her forehead that she was thinking hard. She looked far off when she thought hard but I needed her there.

"It sounds weird," I said.

"You just need time to adjust."

Leaving the clinic with hearing aids for the first time, I noticed that everything had language. The door gasped when it opened. The street flashed and blared with pigeons flapping and crowded city traffic.

Mum could see my widened eyes and tensed shoulders and neck. It scared both of us.

"Raymond?" Her voice sounded stuck in the staticky walkie-talkie sound, like it was part of the wind and the invisible whistling.

"Life?" I asked. "Is it this loud?"

At school, everyone had questions for me. *What's that in your ears?* I didn't want to tell them I was deaf like a ski slope. I would say, "These are my plastic ears."

"What do they do?"

"They help me hear things."

"Like what?"

"Things you can't hear on ski slopes."

Years later, standing in the Historic New Orleans Collection gallery, I thought of my grandfather J.K. Antrobus as I faced a large canvas painting titled *A Plantation Burial,* a striking portrait of a group of black men huddled for a burial. The black preacher man at the center of the painting, with a priest collar and gray curly hair, tilts his head and raises his eyes and hands to the sky as a body is committed to the earth.

In one corner of the painting is a white man with his hand resting on his white horse. At the other end is a couple, a white man and woman in high-society attire, top hat and tuxedo on the man, white puffed-out dress and pearls on the woman. It was painted in 1860, oil on canvas. My co-parent, Tabitha, works as an art conservator and had recently discussed with me some research from conservators at Yale, premised on a rarely seen painting by Bartholomew Dandridge, titled A *Young Girl with an Enslaved Servant and a Dog* (ca. 1725). The painting had spent decades untreated in storage and when retrieved by the conservators they found the darker colors on Dandridge's canvas degraded faster than the rest of the painting, which meant the black figure in the composition had been almost completely obscured.

Tabitha, pointing to all the dark shadows between the cypress trees and the black men on the canvas before us, thought of Dandridge's painting and what we were seeing on the canvas in front of us now. Ruminated on the component that made darker-hued paint and how it was often made with unstable material, meaning many black and darker-skinned people had literally disappeared, vanished from canvases like this one, in which they once appeared. Art conservators over the centuries often missed them, or failed them, the chemicals not keeping them present on the canvas. Many of these darker-skinned figures were only discovered after museums began x-raying more canvases from these periods and finding their ghostly outlines. It's about more than the depiction, but the valuing of the material and a history in need of constant revision.

While peering at the plaque we saw the painter's name. *John Antrobus*. Knowing what my grandmother had told me about the Antrobus name, the village, the way every Antrobus ancestor can be traced to that village, I thought of this while looking at the background of the painting, the pockets of cloudy pink-blue sky through the trees, a just-visible steamboat on the Mississippi River foregrounded by black children resting on the grass playing, oblivious to the weight of the coffin beside them. Antrobus witnessed this scene and left a mark permanent enough for Tabitha and me, his future family, one and a half centuries later, to see it too, to take account of both Tabitha's history and my own.

At my grandma Barbara's funeral the church was packed. Despite outliving all her peers and close friends and most of her relatives, she still created enough connections with the world to fill the congregation. She wasn't rich or famous, never chased recognition. I've been to a lot of funerals since, and it is still the biggest crowd of mourners I've seen. I asked my mother what she lost that day.

"I'm not going to get sentimental about it," she said, crossing her legs, twirling one strand of her gray hair between her fingers. "She was on Earth, gave so much, and now she's gone."

"How do you think she made such an impact in her life?" I asked.

My mother thought for a moment before she spoke.

"She listened to people," she replied, winding another strand of hair tightly around her finger. "People loved her because she listened to them."

4

The Quiet Ear

Searching through the shelves in the secondhand bookstore on Oak Street, uptown New Orleans, I pull out an anthology called *The Quiet Ear*. I flick through and open on a poem by Ted Hughes titled "Deaf School." It's new to me. I read the poem and quietly gasp.

In the early eighties Hughes was commissioned by the National Theatre to research "how people live without language." This idea—that the deaf don't have language, that they live in a world of silence and animalistic gestures rather than the sophistication of speech and canonical literature—compelled him to visit a deaf school in London and observe children learning. His poem uses animal metaphors to describe the movements of the children, two within the first line, "monkey nimble, fish tremulous," then a few lines in the deaf children are "small night lemurs caught in the flash light," "alert," "simple," "lacked a dimension."

Every description positions the speaker of the poem as a wise observer; there's a tone of certainty that pathologizes the deaf children, seeing them as passive amusements.

There's a description of the deaf children's bodies being removed and distant from the air in the room, an idea that they live, simple and "through the eyes," which to me dehumanizes them, not quite as strongly as Joseph Conrad's description of the native Congolese tribe in *Heart of Darkness* as "savages," but it's halfway there.

The biggest irony is that Hughes is lazily describing something highly sophisticated, the language of sign, where meaning is carried in the face and body. He says:

> Their selves were hidden, and their faces looked out of
> hiding.

But Hughes was witnessing empowered deaf children in their own environment, connecting by sign, not hidden by anyone in the room except him.

Hughes is one of the most revered poets in English literature; his collection *The Hawk in the Rain* was one of the first I had read from front to back. In the title poem, the hawk is a noble master whose "wings hold all creation in a weightless quiet," before it is destroyed within its own natural element, despite its power and grace. Seeing Hughes use his poetic gift to frame deaf children as animalistic simpletons was a double assault to me, disappointing and hurtful. What is the use of a poet who uses their talents to enforce harmful stereotypes on marginalized people and their language? I bought the anthology and thought how best to respond to this poem. I needed to meet Hughes at his level: extended metaphors, nature imagery, personification were often his most powerful devices.

Later, sitting by the Mississippi River, feeling the water in the air and the sound of the river in my head, I chose to speak as the river, to speak back to Hughes, a river that could mirror his language back to him. I wrote out each of the descriptions he gave the deaf children and mirrored them back: "Ted was alert and simple, Ted lacked a dimension, Ted lived through his eyes . . ." I struck a line through Hughes's poem and, months later, wanted to publish it in that form. However, as the poem was still legible, I needed permission from the Ted Hughes estate, which they promptly denied. I decided to redact the poem so only its shape remained in thick blacked-out lines, but the journals I submitted it to still refused to publish it. It wasn't until it appeared in my first collection, *The Perseverance,* that the poem found readers.

"Deaf School" by Ted Hughes

After Reading "Deaf School" by the Mississippi River

No one wise calls the river *unaware or simple pools;*
no one wise says it *lacks a dimension;* no one wise
says *its body is removed from the vibration of air.*

The river is a quiet breath-taker, gargling mud.

Ted is *alert* and *simple.*
Ted *lacked a subtle wavering aura of sound*
and responses to Sound.

Ted lived through his eyes. But eye the colossal
currents from the bridge. Eye riverboats
ghosting a geography of fog.

Mississippi means Big River, named by French colonizers.
The natives laughed at their arrogant maps,
conquering wind and marking mist.

The mouth of the river laughs. A man in a wetsuit emerges,
pulls misty goggles over his head. Couldn't see a thing.
He breathes heavily. My face was in darkness.

No one heard him; the river drowned him out.

I once showed this redacted Ted Hughes poem to the students at Knightsfield deaf school in Hertfordshire, after being invited there by Shula, a teacher of the deaf. I held the poem up and asked the students what they saw. A boy at the front with cochlear implants raised his hand. "Sir, turn the page to the side."

I turned it diagonally.

"Now it looks like the sound channels on the screen at my audiologist's when he's programming my implant."

I'll never forget that—a powerful lesson in what creativity can be.

After ironically winning the Ted Hughes Award for my collection *The Perseverance,* I used the prize money to buy new digital hearing aids. Meaning, I came off the NHS and went private. The audiologist who fitted my new hearing aids was surprised when he took my hearing test. He said he sees people with my level of deafness who struggle more visibly with it. A common myth about deaf people is that what we lack in hearing is compensated for with another sense, like a superpower. My superpower has become lip-reading and perfecting my listening face, so it looks like I'm fluidly following speech, nodding, relaxing my shoulders, loosening my jaw. I've found that if you physically express your listening then people open up and talk more, which gives me more time to get used to the voice and speech patterns of a person. These internal gymnastics mean piecing together the things I hear with the missing parts.

But I was born with my deafness and most of a private audiologist's patients are late deafened so it's different. "Physicians in particular, tend to underestimate the quality of life of disabled people, compared with our own assessments of our lives," writes author and disability rights advocate Harriet McBryde Johnson in her essay "Unspeakable Conversations."

I'm not trying to speak to other people's deafness, even though hearing people are constantly speaking to what they think it is. On Hunter Street in central London, I once passed a sign above a shop:

THE I ING OF FALAFEL

The broken parts of the letter "K" that became an "I" reminded me of all the parts of words I don't hear and have to fill in. "The I ing of Falafel" matched my internal deaf dilemma and externalized the language of that internal space, the part of me that is wondering if I heard something correctly and the part of me that is wondering if I've found a poem to perform.

I started to think that a deaf person asserting their relationship to their specific deafness is a necessary kind of performativity. How we perform seems to depend on the audience we're performing for. The Deaf even code-switch among themselves; perhaps speaking with a hard of hearing person is different for a Deaf person, signing without your voice, or using speech and Sign Supported English (SSE), or just lip-reading.

My first collection, *The Perseverance,* had to perform as both a text and a performance, it had to work on the page, and in sign and speech; it's one of the reasons almost all the poems are in a conversational voice. Much of my experience in the hearing world is asking people to repeat themselves; I leaned into the traditional and nontraditional forms of repetition on both page and stage. Repetition in poetry, forms like sestinas, broken ghazals, pantoums, list poems, all of them appear on the page using repeated words and phrases, yet how would I convey this on the stage when I'm speaking to and from the languages of deaf and hearing worlds?

When I work with BSL interpreters on these poems, I emphasize that they can be freer in the location, hand shape, and movement of the signs; they don't need to use the same sign for the repeated parts, they can play and expand the meanings with their sign, like poets who are also translators.

For example, my poem "I Want the Confidence Of" uses the word "confidence" twenty times. "Confidence" is signed in BSL with the "C" hand shape on the lower abdomen raised toward the chest, as if you are lifting the "C" shape toward your heart, but I ask the signers to go further each time it is signed to bring the word further up, to the neck, the throat, the mouth, so by the time I get to the line "I want to be fluent in confidence so large it speaks from its own sky" I want the sign to go above the head and leave the body, entering a new orbit.

As a deaf poet, I avoided writing about my deafness at first, for fear of being simplified and pigeonholed, as if I am only performing for other deaf people, limiting my potential crossover appeal to the mainstream world. Deafness is one part of my identity but the themes I write into—communication, family, education, creativity—aim to have wider appeal.

Now, I feel that a sign of wide acclaim is knowing who we are as deaf people among ourselves, who we are when we turn away from the hearing mainstream gaze altogether; who might we be if we lived in a world of understanding ourselves first, what books could we be writing, what music could we be making, what beats have we been missing, what beats have we been taking, what could we give and take from our most authentic performances?

Institutional deaf education didn't exist in the United Kingdom until the mid-1700s. Before that, only private tutors educated deaf people from noble families. Thomas Braidwood, one of the pioneers of deaf education in the UK, began this way too. Born hearing and from a family of teachers, Braidwood opened the first deaf school in England, in Hackney, east London, in 1783, a mile from my childhood home.

At first he taught literacy but began specializing in deaf education after taking on pupils from rich families who reported improvements in their child's communication skills. Without education, the deaf were cut off from language, community, and society. Many of the early teachers of the deaf were Christian missionaries whose self-prescribed roles were to "save" the deaf, offering them salvation toward Christ through the written, spoken, and sometimes signed word, but this integration required an expertise and deaf awareness that wasn't yet widely developed.

Braidwood's school was called the Academy for the Deaf and Dumb. Notable Deaf students who graduated went on to become barristers, teachers, and governors. Though Thomas Braidwood was Scottish, his reputation grew in England after Dr. Samuel Johnson visited Braidwood's Edinburgh school, where he remarked: "The improvement of Braidwood's pupils is wonderful, they read, write and speak when addressed directly, and distinctly, they lip read so well, it is an expression scarcely figurative to say they hear with the eye."

Braidwood's Academy was a private institution, afforded only by the wealthy; as such, most of the deaf students came from royal and aristocratic families in the UK and its colonies. MP Charles James Fox's deaf son was educated by Braidwood and was written about in the British press as a "remarkable young man who speaks with his fingers." A governor of Barbados educated by Braidwood visited the school whenever he returned to England. Braidwood hadn't intended his academy to function as a private institution, but in the eighteenth century there was not yet legislative or governmental provision for educating the deaf, so he didn't have a choice. Meaning, if you were deaf and wanted an education, you'd better have the money.

American historian and teacher of the deaf Harlan Lane felt that even in the 1990s this was still largely true. "Even now, Deaf education is left to the vagaries of charity and to exploitation by profit seekers."

This legacy of exclusivity continues. Gallaudet University in Washington, DC, is the only university designed for Deaf and hard of hearing students in the world. As of 2024, its annual tuition fee is almost $20,000, which is still a barrier for most, a cost for community, connection, and language.

In 1927, at the age of seven, the South African–born poet David Wright lost his hearing. He was educated at Northampton School for the Deaf in England and often credited his first teacher of the deaf, Miss Neville, and several of his private tutors, as the reason he got into Oxford University in 1939 and for his subsequent success as a poet.

His deafness was a result of a brush with scarlet fever. As Wright lay in his hospital bed recovering from his illness, doctors told his father that his son had lost his hearing, and that it might not return.

Wright's father, sitting by his son's bedside, eyes bloodshot, hands trembling, asked,

Would you like me to read to you?

Wright's father read very well; he had a good baritone voice. He occasionally halted the story he was reading to ask, *Can you hear me now?*

It was a question that confused Wright, but he answered, nodding yes, drowsy and glad as he drifted off to sleep.

Wright then woke in the hospital, his father in his office suit. His father pulled out his gold watch from his pocket and placed it by Wright's ear.

Can you hear it tick?

Wright shook his head, which was covered in thick bandages after being operated on. In the coming weeks the watch experiment became a ritual. Over time, Wright discovered his missing sounds and detailed his struggles in his 1969 autobiography, *Deafness,* one of the most referenced memoirs by a deaf poet in the twentieth century.

The realization of deafness slowly dawned on Wright as he came to in his hospital bed: His mother's voice was becoming an illusion, his eyes were translating sound, voices he had known forever became phantasmal, ghouls, "projections of habit and memory." It was his eyes that diagnosed his deafness, the moment he realized that if he couldn't see his mother's mouth, he couldn't hear her. Wright wasn't afraid or angry; the realization was gradual, his new world was fed to him bit by bit.

Initially, fear, anger, and shame had spared Wright but not his parents. They began their painful speculations about who their child could be now, how would he be educated? What jobs could he take? How would he socialize? They had no idea what liberties and limitations lay ahead for him, no map to dream up their child's future.

"In the case of the deaf child," writes Wright, "it is the parents that do the suffering, at least to begin with. . . . The problem that faced my parents from the moment I lost my hearing had been my education." Wright's parents were hearing. Wright's father was wealthy enough to afford private tutors.

Wright was late deafened; my deafness was discovered late. I assumed before reading Wright's autobiography that our experience, especially our education and work life, would be distinguishable. It wasn't. The overlaps are sharp and acute.

Before I reread my childhood journals, I assumed I'd denied my deafness until I was in my early twenties, but it wasn't true. In a diary entry dated September 15, 1998, I was desperate to assert that I struggled to hear. I wrote in long, wonky, misspelled sentences that I wasn't understood as a deaf person, that *I really can't hear and no one seems to be adjusting to my needs*, that *people think I'm faking because of the way I speak*, that *I don't look deaf.*

A later entry, in January 2000, at fourteen years old, I wrote about a girl I liked and the reasons she'd reject me: *being deaf doesn't suit me.*

By the winter of 1928, Wright's family fled South Africa for England, seeking advice from specialists and teachers of the deaf. Wright would shuffle through the freeze of London and the parks of Kensington Gardens, and skate on the frozen lake by the Serpentine. He would stroll with friends past Buckingham Palace to read the bulletins of the king's declining health posted on the railings.

With his dulled hearing, Wright wandered through the vibrating city, absorbing the visual patchwork of the bustle, the concrete mishmash of dialogue with time and place. London's smoky streets blared with Victorian gaslit lampposts that ran along cobblestone pavements. Roman roads rumbled with iron trams, Oxford Street burst with open-topped double-decker buses, square, squat taxicabs, and bicycles, all bobbed with bowler-hatted or cloth-capped men. Some Tudor houses had Georgian windows, some stylish streets of Art Deco houses stood beside redbrick Edwardian terraces.

Yet, it was the railings that defined the city for Wright, railings that wrapped around parks, gardens, palaces, cathedrals, hospitals, churchyards, memorials, houses, pubs—standing *stoosh* (as my father would say in patois) to mark and claim the territory.

In the specialist Ear, Nose and Throat Hospital on Harley Street in central London, Wright's father listened to the sales talk of suited specialists who drained his bank balance on consultations and rang tuning forks behind his son's ears, syringed oils into his canals, laid him on couches, clubbed parts of his vertebrae, pumped soapy water up his rectum, and strapped electrical pads around his ears (which left him jittery after an accidental electrocution). Wright described it as hellish but also a testament to his parents' "love and despair."

After all the efforts in England failed, Wright returned to Johannesburg for a last-resort visit to a faith healer, a short, elderly "well-to-do woman" who lived in a large, white-brick house facing a neat, blossoming square patch of garden. The self-professed spirit medium stirred her hands for hours in the air above Wright's head. He sat pensively in a polished oakwood chair.

After a year, still deaf, his speech began to blur. His parents, having thrown whatever money they could at the stubborn walls of Wright's deafness, began to accept the reality of it. This meant managing his remaining hearing and speech with a teacher of the deaf.

Wright returned to London later in 1928, this time to the pillared arches of Regent's Park Crescent. Here they were introduced to Miss Neville, a silver-haired, straight-backed woman with Edwardian elegance who taught privately. Wright credited her as the founder of his education, the teacher who "rescued me from inarticulateness," rounding out his speech with enunciation exercises and tightening his cursive handwriting and mathematical skills. There was only one other student, a slightly older girl called Vanessa. They were taught orally, without sign.

In Miss Neville's first lesson Wright was ordered to stand up and repeat vowels, individually, then together, slow then fast:

Say E

E

Say A

A

Now say E A

E A

Say S

S

Now say them all together

E A S

Very good, repeat
E A S
Faster
E A S, E A S, E A S
E A S, E A S, yes
(Wright unconsciously says yes)

There you are, John (Wright's birth name was John; he later changed it to David), *you can say yes perfectly.*

These types of "speech drills"—endlessly repeating a litany of monosyllables—helped Wright unlock parts of his tongue, pronouncing the fuller sound of vowels and consonants.

Vanessa was the first deaf child Wright had met, "fair haired with a stony expression," and as articulate and neat as Wright but with what he called a "strangely limited" general knowledge. Vanessa did not know the name of the king of England in class, stating "King United Kingdom," whereupon Wright shook his head, puffed up his chest, and launched the answer:

"King George the Fifth!"

Miss Neville nodded approvingly.

Wright noted that Vanessa's vocabulary was more limited than his, having been born deaf, and she had a harder time acquiring words from spoken conversation and random reading. Wright realized his advantages in Miss Neville's oralist method lessons as a late-deafened person who already had the foundation of speech, though he would never acknowledge the disadvantages of not learning sign language.

Wright wrote his first verses after reading Kipling and an Edwardian selection of poetry. What most enthused him was the tune, music he could extract from metered lines. Wright had a fondness for music and had played the violin before going deaf.

In some way poetry substituted for his playing practice—he was now scoring with language, saying he would not have "troubled [his] head with the stuff [poetry]" if it wasn't for his deafness.

I have as many alignments as I do contentions with Wright. Wright wrote cynically about deaf empowerment. He calls *What the Mind Hears* by Harlan Lane—one of the most significant books written on the history of Deaf education—"tenacious propaganda for sign language." He thought lip-reading and finger-spelling couldn't be considered elegant and that a deaf person cannot be complete without integration into the hearing world.

"Deaf people ought to not have too much to do with each other . . ." said Wright, a startling sentence that he quickly qualifies. "Yet, it is only the deaf who can teach the deaf how to live."

I believe Wright lived his whole life with deaf shame, perhaps internalized his parents' anxieties as a newly deafened child, with the barriers he faced being deaf in a hearing world shaming him too deeply. Between the lines in his autobiography, Wright never seems to find stability and harmony between these two worlds, and this resonated with a younger version of myself more than half a century after he wrote it.

Wright changed his name when he left Northampton School for the Deaf, from John to David, which he described as a "symbolic exorcism of my deaf persona."

The poems he wrote in his youth wouldn't mention his deafness—he wanted to disappear from his body and into pure pronounceable language like the railings and pillared arches that defined the heart of London, his preferred city.

It is in the poem "On Himself" in his second collection,

Moral Stories (1954), where Wright allows himself a moment of deaf disclosure.

> Abstracted by silence from the age of seven,
> Deafened and peened by black calamity
> As twice to be born, I cannot without pity
> Contemplate myself as an infant

The etymological root of the word "infant" is "incapable of speech," yet Wright continues to doubt his language ability even beyond his youth. All poets ought to think deeply about the limits of words, whether or not they are colored by the questionable image of "black calamity," implying misfortune and depression.

Shame, shame.

Wright feared failure but not as much as he resented pity. He didn't want to be read as disabled. He operated and flourished in the hearing world of Oxford, abruptly stopping his autobiography after leaving school, stating deafness had nothing to do with his time beyond that because he'd severed almost all contact with the deaf world.

Shame, shame.

In 1992 Wright published "An Appearance of Success," a poem that appears in his last collection. It charts his perspective on receiving public acclaim as a poet after being published on posters on the London Underground and having a widely watched BBC documentary made about his life.

In the poem he addresses his father, wishing he could assert his value to him now that the burden of his deafness could translate into something celebratory.

This present
I'd love to give him to make amends . . .
an appearance of success in his deaf difficult son
something to recompense
as may have seemed to him
rewardless.

In his 1963 speech delivered to the Association of Psychiatric Social Workers, Donald Winnicott states that even as it causes suffering, depression has value as it is bound up with "our discovery of a personal identity." Winnicott implies that if children are able to manage the stresses of depression they may be rewarded with greater self-knowledge and "the achievement of emotional growth."

When the American writer and comedian Drew Michael revealed on the *WTF with Marc Maron* podcast interview that he is deaf (he refers to it as "the hearing thing"), it had me sitting stock-still, the first time I'd heard someone find words for something so similar to my own early experience of deafness. Michael discloses that he is in therapy; he sounds jittery and unsettled, like a man thinking of throwing himself into a lake.

Because of the hearing thing I can't do the whole sit on the couch while the therapist is behind you. If I can't see you, like I can't see your mouth, it's very hard for me to understand what you're saying . . . I have hearing aids but it's not perfect . . .

Michael explains how desperate he was to appear "normal," to not want to be a "burden" to his parents.

Like Wright and Michael, in my early years I wished away

my deafness, refused sign language, stayed loosely connected to the deaf world in the background bushes, attuned myself, pretended I could hear when I couldn't, overcompensated and overexplained, cautious of pity and tokenism, wanting to be liked and recognized on merit, which meant blending in, hiding my deafness, not publishing poems that signposted my identities, wanting to stay aloof and pass. If I ask people to repeat, or I tick the disabilities box on that form, if I wear both hearing aids I look disabled not desirable, if I take too long to answer questions I'm failing, the girl will reject me, the public will pity me, they will act awkward, assume me slow.

Shame, shame. It seemed to follow me everywhere.

When I was seven, Wright's age, I wasn't yet at a deaf school but I did benefit from a teacher of the deaf. At my school, the playground was on the roof, which was like a huge concrete square with tall plastic mesh fencing around it. It now looked to me like a net filled with new sounds. I heard a lot more of the sky. The wind had a new temper, planes sounded like they were falling or flying too close to the ground, birds were constant and mad and full of panicky songs.

AHHHIIIIIII

I looked up at the sky.

AHHHHIIIIII

Were ghosts whistling?

I looked at my feet and my hands; there was no way to tell what direction each sound came from.

AHHHIIIIIII

It sounded far away.

I saw a girl running.

AHHHHIIIIII!

Carly, a girl in my class, was holding her hairband—it had come loose as she ran.

AHHHHIIIIII

Was she being chased?

AHHHIII!

I ran over to the far end of the playground near the drinking fountains. *AHHHIII!* A boy was behind her. Camillo. He was holding something cupped in his hands. *What happened?* Camillo opened his hand like the lid of a precious case. A frog.

Small, green in his palm. Croaking. Another new sound.

Where did you find that?

Camillo pointed at the drain by the drinking fountain, which was dripping and sounded like it was thinking.

My teacher Mr. Barry started treating me differently. He looked at me more in class. He became even friendlier. When he was reading a book, he asked me to sit by his feet. Every time he looked up from the book he glanced directly at me to make sure I was following the story. I liked Mr. Barry because he was really good at pulling funny faces and making voices, especially while reading stories.

Because Mr. Barry was so good at making faces he said a lot without words. He had a face that said, *Are you listening?* Another look that said, *Copy what I write on the board,* and one that said, *I am worried about you.*

I remember wondering why Mr. Barry seemed worried about me. I wondered if he was keeping me close because he could hear things that weren't there.

In class Mr. Barry stood next to Renata. She had glasses and brown-grayish hair, looking like an owl in a cardigan. I had met Renata once; she came into class and said she was going to observe me. She was the second teacher of the deaf that I had met. It was her job to help me develop language and communication skills. As I was in a hearing school, it was her responsibility to ensure I assimilated into the mainstream hearing world.

She sat in the corner with a clipboard. Afterward she took me into a room I'd never been in before. It had a sofa and cushions and the radiator was on even though it was warm outside. She asked if I liked school, and then she said some words and asked me to repeat them after her. Then she said some different words but this time with a piece of paper over her mouth. She had a habit of nodding, giving the exact same reaction to anything I repeated, giving me no clues if I was getting them right. Afterward she put down the paper and showed me I'd got some words right but some words wrong. Maybe today she was going to test the whole class?

"Hello, class, I'm here to talk about things we hear and things some of us don't hear and why." Renata held up a picture of an ear but there were lots of shapes and parts on it that you can't see because those parts are inside your head.

I had seen the same picture in the serious doctor's clinic. The feeling of knowing something no one else did was like electricity because it lit up my body and made my heart pound because I might at last be right about something.

A boy in class calmly raised his hand. "It's a diagram of an ear."

"Good." Renata pointed to different parts of the ear like they were different rooms in a spaceship: the cartilage, the ear canal, the earlobe, the eardrum, and then the "inner ear." Then she pointed to something that looked like a shell with a spiral pattern. Once, I picked up a shell while walking on a beach with my mother. "Put your ear to the shell and hear the sea," said Mum. But I put my ear to it and heard nothing.

"This is the cochlea," said Renata. "It's our inner radio and needs to be tuned in for us to hear properly. We have little hairs in our ears that pick up sound and these are our aerials that carry sound to the cochlea.

"The strength of our signals can be different for different people." Renata put down the diagram. "Like Raymond."

The heat of every ear in the class on me made me sweat.

"Raymond needs devices in his ears to help strengthen his hearing."

Carly had a look of disgust on her face.

"There might even be things that Raymond can hear now that some of you can't."

I could hear the walkie-talkie static of the air and the nerves in my head and chest like a large wave about to crash.

Camillo raised his hand. "Can Raymond hear what we're thinking?"

Everyone looked at me again. Attention is a hot tray, you have to know how to hold it, but I dropped it on the floor with my stammering.

"Um . . . I don't know," I said.

Renata looked at me before she spoke again; her face was asking, *Do you want to speak for yourself?*

I shook my head. *No.*

Mr. Barry raised his hand.

"Renata, I would like to ask the rest of the class a question. Are we going to treat Raymond any differently than we did before?"

I could feel the thinking in the air. A few voices said "Yes" and some said "No."

Mr. Barry said, "Noooo."

Truth is, not even I knew how to answer Mr. Barry's question. Should people treat me differently? I preferred the way my mum talked to me when she was inside the Donald Winnicott Centre exactly because she treated me differently, changing (but only slightly) how she spoke to me, louder, slower, with face-to-face contact. At the same time, I didn't want to be different from anyone else. I wanted to blend in, be "normal." Terms like "differently abled" feel as condescending as "special." Anything that marked difference would make me stand out and standing out made you a target, especially for the boys who were looking for victims, people to pick on. There were some rough kids in the school, boys in gangs, most notably Packington, a group of mainly white English kids, many of whose parents were also in gangs. We knew each of their names, avoided them if we saw them on the canal paths on the way home or resting on the climbing frame in the adventure playground. I had already noticed that my race was another thing that marked me, offered the potential for different treatment. On the gravel football pitch outside the school, an older boy, probably twelve years old with hazel-brown hair in curtains and wearing a gray hoodie, approached and accused me of *not looking English.* A friend, who I suppose looked more English, had to defend me. *Nah, his dad is*

Jamaican and his mum is English. The boy turned to me, pointing a finger in my face. *Is you English or Jamaican?*

English! I said, missing no beat.

The first time I drew a self-portrait I sat next to my friend Paul in class and watched him circle his head and scratch in his hair. I watched Paul color himself pink then asked him if I could borrow his color. Even though I wore hearing aids I never drew them on. They hadn't integrated into my sense of self, and with no deaf peers to mirror my deafness back to me, it stayed out of my self-perception, even as I was putting hearing aids into my ears every day. I had no stable view of my race either, but I picked up on the anxiety my racial ambiguity caused others and played into whatever perception kept me safest; black, white, whatever they wanted to see.

After that, Renata came to my school more often. She took me out of class and sat with me in a small room with one round table in the middle of it. Outside the window, leaves and branches reached through and around the glass as if peering in to wave; I could see the canal, the paths, and the ducks.

I remember Renata's large circular glasses and her constant half smile that was a mix of stoicism and kindness. Her voice was firm, clear, earthy, and because of her precise natural enunciation, she was easy to lip-read. Despite her professional distance I didn't feel like I was being assessed; I felt she was trying to understand me. After each of our sessions she'd write a list of words that she had noticed I hadn't heard and she'd show them to me on her paper. She would look at my writing then write another list of words that I had misspelled or written wrongly. I wrote words as I heard them. A silent sound unstressed in a word was always a hole. For example, "talisman" I spelled "talman," "from" I spelled "rom," "fright" I spelled "right," the "th," "ch," "fa" sounds always eluded my ear, but the sounds I got right were the words I recognized on Renata's list from books and comics I used to read (mainly *Goosebumps* and *The Beano*), words that are spelled exactly how they sound, mainly onomatopoeic words. Oink, meow, bang, splash, beep, plop, these sounds always announce themselves, but all the other words with those silent letters (lasagna, ballet, aisle, psalm, etc.) had a sound that would never be mine and I will always be speaking at the edge of them.

Renata didn't underline or fill my page with red marks; she corrected my mistakes on her own piece of paper in neutral black, blue, or green ink. She went through each sound of the letters and wrote them out, had me focus on the lip pattern as well as the spelling.

That first session she concentrated on the letter "y" because I kept writing it the wrong way. I drew it like a twisted twig. "Y" was difficult because it makes three different sounds depending on where it occurs in a word. For example, the "yeh" in "yellow" is different from the "why" sound in "shy," which is different again from the "ie" sound in "happy."

I couldn't write "y" because I couldn't hear to understand it, so she said to imagine a stick with two arms in the air—*if it appears at the end of a word like "nappy" it makes a long "e" sound*—and she showed me each phonetic sound and lip shape as well as the written word.

Somehow, I never dreaded this reveal of what I had missed or got wrong. She would show me the corrected words and say, "Try to remember this for next time." When I saw her the following week she would begin by asking what I remembered from the last session and recap each of my previous mistakes and then ask me to spell the words.

I think of Renata as one of the fixers of my language, filling holes and showing me the shapes and sensations of tongue and sound. She went above and beyond, cared for me, even showing me how to join up my wonky handwriting while explaining how the English language hides some of its sounds. She thoroughly tracked my progress and kept challenging me with literacy and lip-reading.

All these lessons happened in private, away from the witness of the other schoolchildren: It felt like I was a machine that had to be taken out of the main factory space for specialized maintenance. This didn't bother me; I looked forward to Renata's lessons and never felt like I was less in any way for needing them.

The most memorable smile Renata gave me was when I spelled "physical" correctly. This was after years of her care, when I had shown that I could distinguish the "y" sounds, picking them up even in the middle of a word.

"Intelligent," she said, writing it down. "That's *you*."

Fourteen years after leaving Blanche Nevile deaf school, I found myself back in a classroom learning British Sign Language from Deaf teachers. Deborah, my first teacher of the deaf as an adult, was a standout presence. With her fluid sign and relaxed shoulders, she held herself lightly in stark contrast to the tightness of my body.

She gestured to me that she was "turning off her voice" and signed with me on that first day. I loosely followed and managed by using some of the alphabet and signs that I remembered but all in English word order (Sign Supported English). Encouragingly, she held out her fingers and palm on one hand and clutched an invisible brush with the other hand and brushed each finger as if she was polishing a shoe to gesture that she'd polish up my signs.

Even as an adult, learning BSL didn't securely integrate all parts of my identity but it did help me reconnect with the deaf community and a part of myself that I had spent so long running away from.

I sought out a therapist who specialized in trauma and "relationship construction." When we met online, he would face me through the screen. I recounted my experience at primary and secondary school, processing some of the visceral feelings of that time, feeling unseen, unheard, and within months my angry knots began loosening. Captions flashed across the screen as he spoke:

"Did you feel alone in your story?" he asked, tilting his head back, a stack of David Wright's books in view on the shelf behind me.

"Have you found a new language for yourself?"

5

Choosing My Lane

Between the ages of five and twelve my name appeared on two registers: first at Sharks Swimming Club in Bethnal Green, then at Haggerston Baths in Hackney. It seemed that as long as my body was in the water, my name never disappeared.

At first I was a bystander. My mother took my older sister to the same swimming club, and for years I had to sit in the stands watching her swim, sweating and angsty from the stuffy chlorine heat, until I concluded I might as well follow my sister into the water.

We are all deaf underwater to a certain extent. I felt liberated beneath the surface, the warbling, smeary underwater incoherence, the soft crashing of other bodies joining you in the water, the submerged shimmering atmosphere that enveloped me, as if in a different, more generous dimension that took some of the stiff robotic weight I moved with on the street and around school. I was fluid in my body in a way I wasn't on land.

By the time I was ten I was taking time trials and being entered into national swimming competitions. I wasn't exceptional at a national level, though; my highest average placing was fourth, my strongest stroke, butterfly.

Butterfly is the most dramatic and strenuous of all the strokes. Arms strive, push, propel the body through the surface, the breath is gulped, the kicks flop, bob, and pound like a mermaid.

I was built for this stroke, although I remember a boy at the time saying, *You're cut, but you have a body like a cereal box,* so he always called me "Shreddies." Regardless, I am naturally slender with wide shoulders that launch the rest of my body; kicks, glide, gasping, all of it leaves a choppy trail of disturbed foamy waves.

My swimming coach at Haggerston pool was called Mark. Despite being in his early thirties, he appeared like a twenty-year-old, like a baby-faced member of a nineties boy band—Mark Owen from Take That, probably. Light brown curtained hair, small broody hazelnut eyes, and (usually) clean-shaven, he always wore white shorts no matter the weather or setting. His voice was deeper than you'd expect from his appearance: deep, clear. He was a confident and gifted communicator.

It would be easy to see Mark as a stand-in for my (part-time, often unreliable) father—a man I needed attention from when it was lacking elsewhere. But this would be an unhelpful and most likely untrue trope. It is true, though, that throughout my teens and early twenties, the people I latched onto, wanting their attention and approval, were men.

Everyone in the swimming group liked Mark; he was funny,

friendly, and encouraging. I swam as long as I did because of his presence. I had developed, privately, an emotional investment in wanting his attention and approval; I longed to impress him, to be seen by him.

Mark gave patient and observant demonstrations. He would stand on the poolside gesturing proper form, guiding you through techniques. He was good at mimicking the faults in your form, then correcting them through physical demonstration with a focused vocabulary of verbs and images:

enter water here,
become an eel, a dolphin
a carved canoe,
fingertip first, here—
Tree shape, here,
circular, here
tree trunk, here,
scoop water, slide, turtle fin, here
elbow out, not like a frog,
like a gliding wave approaching
the shore, sync feet, knees
and mermaid kick,
butterfly,
strive . . .

Mark knew I was deaf. I started swimming with him the year I got hearing aids. At the start of the sessions he had all the swimmers huddled in a close circle; he'd ensure I was standing next to him (I could keep my hearing aids in this way), and he'd calmly, loudly speak the routines from the poolside. Once I was in the water and my hearing aids were out, he'd give instructions standing above my lane.

If he saw I was struggling he'd tell me to get out so he could speak to me directly. He repeated everything, moves and words, at least three times. His voice would boom brightly, so despite what was lost in the holes of indoor pool heat and chlorine, I listened and learned with my eyes, following the expressions of his body.

I felt seen and unseen by Mark. I was a middle-ability swimmer in the high-achieving ranks of the club. I never got any special attention: He was equally kind and encouraging to all his swimmers. To do well, you had to show up, train toward your time trials, beat your previous times, and then try to qualify for the nationals. The system had no space for favoritism or subjectivity: You either qualified or you didn't.

You only knew who his favorites were (as swimmers) at the annual award ceremonies. The sting of not being acknowledged at any of the ceremonies grew each year. Most promising swimmer, most improved, most dedicated, most awarded medals—

Once, while we were gathered in a circle on the poolside, I desperately needed a piss, but Mark was in full swing, going over our stroke routines: "four lengths front crawl, backstroke, breaststroke, watch the turns" . . . The sixty-second clock spun its yellow hands on the wall behind him as I decided to let it all out; no one would notice, they're all watching Mark, we are wet from the pool, it'll run invisibly down my leg, who will see? No one.

Without looking down I stayed focused on Mark's mouth while I unleashed a full, fast stream of piss. It took a few seconds for Mark to stop speaking and look at me; some of the swimmers followed Mark's eyes. Mark cleared his throat. One of the girls, a club champion, tapped her friend and pointed at me; I remember tensing my six-pack in case that's what they were looking at, but both scrunched up their faces like used tissues. *Ew,* I heard, then looked down. I wore skintight Speedo trunks; my dehydrated dark brown-yellow piss laser-beamed from my tip through my trunks. My piss pooled around the feet of every swimmer. I gasped quietly.

To this day I have flashbacks of this moment; it cramps my stomach still, pulsing through the top part of my abdominals, like a red fish squirming below my ribs. My body hasn't forgotten it. The finger point, the scrunched face, Mark's brief pause, even the yellow hand on the wall is damp and stuck. Even though it's more than likely that everyone who witnessed it has forgotten that image, the piercing shame of it is an enduring alarm, a fat unblinking fish out of water.

I got changed thinking of something my sister had said to me once . . .

"Raymond, you're not slick or sly," she said, holding the CD I'd stolen from her room, my fingerprints glaring off it, the case it came in cracked. "Never try to commit a crime, because it's you, you'll be caught."

My first swimming event on the national stage was in Derby. I was the youngest in my race by a few years. I stood on the starter block, one foot forward, one back. Everyone's head was down; mine was to the side so I could see the starter pistol, afraid I'd react too late to the sound. I leaped from my block—my dive wasn't neat: I dove down, deep, rather than glide, skim straight into the water. It was a weak start. I surfaced and scooped, kicked, tumble-turned, and pushed away from the wall at the far end after the first length, but the gap it put between myself and the other swimmers never shortened. I came in last. Humiliated, I climbed out of the pool and ran to the changing rooms, crying.

As we got on the coach back to London, Mark put his hand on my shoulder. "We need to work on your starts. You're slow off the block, you dive too deep, but once you start your stroke you're stronger." This consoled me; it was practical advice, it softened my negative self-talk, shifted it from my personal feelings of inferiority to the inferiority of the performance and how it could be improved. It was also proof that Mark had seen me and cared.

In the swimming lessons the following week Mark had the starter blocks screwed into the poolside floor. I dove and dove, too deep, too deep. Mark, running thin on patience but not giving up, decided to take off his shirt and shoes and get into the pool himself. He angled himself straight, a sharp missile, his feet connecting with the water so he could glide forward, arms stretched out in front of him, and began his stroke. It was such a smooth dive that my mind recorded it; I still visualize it before diving into a pool.

In fact, my mind has recorded a lot of Mark, his demonstrations, his firm, encouraging voice. His voice is a constant companion in the water: *scoop—kick—glide—slice—tumble—push—push—push*. His catalogue of verbs keeps me moving between the walls of water, has me finishing with one hand on the wall from the front crawl, the backstroke, both hands from the butterfly, the breaststroke, lifting my head toward the clock. I hear Mark—*you need to shave four seconds from that time.* Mark is present, physically pushing me to make it.

After my second year at the nationals, improving but not achieving a high rank (I came in seventh), then not being acknowledged at the end-of-year ceremony, despite these improvements, I quit. I was thirteen.

Triad, a gang that operated in north London snooker clubs, had recruited a friend of mine, and they asked him to recommend someone who was fit and fast for a job. I was put forward and recruited to deliver parcels in council estates around King's Cross and Angel. I was given the parcels (either brown or white), thickened by the Sellotape wrapped around them, and left them outside doors or under stairways to be picked up. I was never told what was in the parcels, but I was paid £50 a day.

The man who recruited me was a Chinese man, probably mid-twenties, dressed head to toe in white. He had dark cropped hair and spoke in fast, abrupt sentences in broken English. I first met him with my friend outside the snooker hall. "This is him," said my friend.

"Hey, yes, you fast, yeah?"

I nodded.

"Good."

As we were standing on the street two boys came walking past us; one of them made eye contact with the Triad member. "Hey, what you look at . . . ?" said the Triad member, raising his head, sticking out his chest, then yelling, "Chief!" The boy looked away, knowing he was being challenged but choosing to walk on.

A few years ago I gave a poetry workshop in a maximum-security men's prison. One of the men told me he had started out his criminal life delivering packages when he was eleven years old. I asked if he knew what was in them. He said he didn't at the time, but later found out it was heroin, cocaine, and ecstasy pills. Realizing I was likely delivering drugs too made me realize how lucky I was not to have been in prison myself. I also felt guilt for the harm caused to desperate people, but I was a child—there was so much I didn't know.

After a year I stopped working for Triad because the friend who had recruited me had gone into a witness protection program after he tried to leave the gang. Triad wanted to make him a permanent member. His initiation into the gang was to stab someone but he refused. Triad turned on him and beat him unconscious. I saw him when he came out of the hospital, the deep bruising looked like someone had painted a map of black and purple countries on his face and neck. His black eyes had only just healed enough for him to open them.

My friend boasted that when you walk around with black eyes, visible bruises, no one messes with you because it's proof that you aren't afraid to fight. "You can't handle this," said my friend. "You better lay low."

I remembered thinking that the main reason I didn't want black eyes was because of the questions my dad might ask about them. "Rah tid!" he'd say. "What'appen, your face bruck nuh, tell me yuh mash up dem boys who did dat deh?"

His concern wouldn't be as much the pain inflicted on me as the pain I was capable of inflicting on "dem boy deh." I would have to show or say that I didn't go down without a fight, and the truth is, in some of my fights I had allowed the other boy to win (because he had an older brother or a gang that backed him that would have come for me if I didn't).

My dad never found out about Triad. He didn't even know I'd stopped swimming. He was neutral about me swimming in the first place; it was more that I had somewhere to be and something to do that he liked. He'd say it was good that I wasn't getting mixed up with the foolishness of the boys on the streets.

I didn't have to worry him with my Triad involvement because they didn't know where we lived. I was savvy enough to know the territories Triad operated in and avoid them, so I could stay in my lane.

Recently, my mother found pictures of me at twelve, fourteen, and sixteen. I look at those faces and I don't recognize those boys now. Even my partner, looking at the photos, says, "My God, you've been ten different people."

After Triad, I returned to swimming, craving the safety and familiarity of the pool, a depth I could handle, but it wasn't the same. I struggled to keep up with the swimmers I used to share the lane with. As they glided past me, I was confused by the pulsing feeling in my stomach and chest. Fatigue: I'd never felt like that before. I thought it was something attacking my body: a lizard, perhaps, something heavy with slime and heat.

My year out of the pool was the year I was caught smoking weed at school and sent home. I thought my dad was going to beat me when he found out, but he chuckled and said, "Ray, listen, the stuff you get on the streets is no good," and he showed me a marijuana plant. "This is homegrown—promise me you won't smoke the skunk or chemical street stuff and I'll give you my homegrown." I kept that promise, but also started using tobacco because the leaves burned down too quickly on their own.

In the pool I realized that was the lizard in my body. I asked my arms, legs, and chest why they were stiffer, slower; I asked my muscles why they were burning.

At school, though, I was one of the strongest swimmers. I was made captain of my swim team, won multiple races, took the swim team to glory. A popular girl in school, K, started noticing me and asked me out. I said yes, not because I felt any way about her, but because of the look some of the other boys gave me when they found out the popular girl liked me—a mix of surprise and jealousy. Did male attention and approval always mean more to me? I think it did. I think I had internalized ideas of masculinity that were stiff and toxic; I think the kind of boy I was trying to be was physically tough and emotionally numb, the paradox of course being these are the traits of psychopaths.

In a scene from an early episode of *The Fresh Prince of Bel-Air,* Will Smith tries to show his niece Ashley how to fight. "You got to show them you're crazy . . . hey, hey, back up, back up, mind your business okay, just mind your business." The joke is that to survive the playground bullies you had to maintain and dramatize an aura of danger and violent capability; you had to make people think you were crazy, wild, unpredictably violent; backing down and refusing the metrics of conventional, straight male masculinity wasn't an option.

My dad enforced this logic with his own unpredictable violence and rages. Once, he told me he was set on by an Irish man who knocked him unconscious outside a pub, but the man ended up picking him up off the floor and buying him a drink, respecting him for just being willing to fight.

Back at school, once the shine and glory of winning the school swimming tournament wore off, K sent her friend over to dump me. "K says you're dumped because you keep ignoring her." I was baffled. "She says hello and you keep blanking her."

But I wasn't blanking K. I couldn't hear her voice. It was too soft. I tried to explain.

"She doesn't care, it's done."

Most people in the UK won't have heard of the Deaflympics but it is one of the oldest multi-sporting events in the world. In 1924 it was launched as the "International Silent Games," thirty-six years before the Paralympics began in 1960.

During my years as a swimmer, I never heard of the Deaflympics. Deaflympic swimmer Nathan Young, ranked fifth in the world in a number of Deaflympic events and winner of a bronze medal in 2017 representing Great Britain, makes the case that Deaflympic swimmers don't get funded by the main funding body, Swim England, and he has relied on his parents and personal fundraising campaigns to support his swimming career. He wants to correct this situation so that deaf swimmers can compete fairly, with proper sponsorship and support.

When he wrote to Swim England asking about the lack of financial support, he was told: "Swim England does not receive funding for talent development for deaf swimmers because the pathway does not lead to Paralympic events."

"How on earth did someone come up with the idea that deaf athletes should not be funded but someone with a learning difficulty or blindness should be?" ponders Young.

I wouldn't have been deaf enough to qualify for the Deaflympics, as they measure the ear with the stronger hearing (my right ear), which has to be fifty decibels or less. I miss the mark by fifteen decibels, meaning, in this context, my lane and all my competitions are with hearing swimmers.

Deaf swimmers like Young are in different lanes and races but still have to compete with hearing swimmers as well as disabled swimmers in the nationals, many of whom are fully funded because they are competing to qualify for the Olympics or the Paralympics. But because the Deaflympics aren't covered by mainstream media, it makes it harder or impossible to be funded by Swim England.

"Money keeps speaking, keeps corrupting our value systems," is what I say as I glimpse a headline today about a Tory MP (Rishi Sunak) who voted to defund a public swimming pool the same week he had a private pool built in his house.

There was one other black boy in the swimming group, Tayo, a Yoruba name meaning "boy full of happiness." The year I came back to swimming, he began picking on me. First muttering "gay," "dumb," "pussy"—words it took me a while to register because of my hearing. My default expression when someone said something I didn't hear was to smile and nod, which wound him up more until the insults became louder, more intense. He started saying them closer to my face.

Do you lick-a-dick-a-day?

Huh?

Only-gays-say-what.

What?

I was so baffled by Tayo's random insults that I couldn't assert myself and interact with him properly. Yet, he continued to mark me, the only other black boy. But he probably didn't know my race; my father never picked me up from swimming so he would have only seen my mother. We were both twelve-year-olds, and it was the year 2000—the year of the Sydney Olympics and Eric the Eel, the only black swimmer I'd ever seen on TV. I watched him on the TV in my dad's council flat on Laburnum Street.

Eric the Eel was a wild card, representing Equatorial Guinea. His real name is Eric Moussambani, and his fame was almost drowning in front of 17,500 spectators watching in the stadium and millions watching around the world, including my dad and me, who were chanting at the TV, "Come on, black man, come on!" as if we all had backed and bet our life savings on him.

The only other two competitors in his heat were disqualified for false starts. The Eel, who had never swum in an Olympic-size pool (only at the beach, in rivers, and in a twenty-meter hotel pool), was left with empty lanes and had only to finish the race to win. It was victory or nothing.

His dive off the block wasn't bad, slow, but smooth enough; he didn't dive too deep. Soon, though, the Eel huffs, burns, pants, he almost sinks, his head barely above water. The audience screams, shouts, the cloud of stadium noise propels the Eel; the sound seeps in and electrifies his body. He finishes, only just.

The moment steals the entire Olympic Games and remains,

to many, the most memorable sporting event of that year. For me, it was complicated, playing me back to that toxic myth about melanin and black people who can't swim. I was learning, when I was twelve, that myths like that came from racist sources such as the American South, where enslaved black people on plantations weren't taught to swim in case it helped them escape, but Eric the Eel affirmed all the negatives.

Which was very unfair. Eric was a real athlete without any training facilities. Four years after his famous race, he was still swimming and planning to take part in the 2004 Olympics in Athens. He had acquired sponsorship from Coca-Cola and Speedo, but it all disappeared due to passport issues. Eric had become a proficient athletic swimmer in the interim. By 2006 he was clocking up times that would have given him gold medals if he had been racing in any 200m Olympic freestyle event between 1896 and 1968, but he was never given the opportunity to show the world how much he had improved.

Today Eric lives in his birthplace town of Malabo, the capital city of Equatorial Guinea. The country now has two Olympic-size swimming pools and Eric, as well as working at a petroleum company, is a swimming coach. In this role he has channeled his Olympic fame into inspiring other athletes from his country, a country that has yet to produce another Olympic swimmer. Eric still dreams of his swimmers delivering gold, but, despite Black American swimmers Cullen Jones (2008, 2012) and Simone Manuel (2016) winning gold, Eric's own appearance as "The Eel" remains to many people the only image of a black Olympic swimmer.

If Tayo had internalized the racist ideas of swimming to prove he was as good (as human) and as worthy as white swimmers, maybe he didn't know I was mixed black, maybe it didn't matter, maybe, to him, I was just different in the wrong way? Perhaps Tayo was projecting, perhaps he was a dickhead. Either way, Eric the Eel affirmed the (white) idea that there could only be one lane for black boys and we'd better stick to it.

I don't know what happened to Tayo. The last time I saw him he'd snarled something aggressively homoerotic. *Suck dick!*

I packed my bag on the changing-room benches, carefully, knowing I wouldn't be returning.

I don't know what happened to Mark after he left the club but every time I swim, he appears in my mind.

He's on the poolside demonstrating a stroke, catching each wonky part of my form, pretending to stick his elbow out of the water,

not here,

closing his elbow closer to his body, straightening it,

here,

let this finger be the first to enter the water.

The Mark in my mind doesn't age; he's like a deity, a saint, a spirit, something static, eternal, ageless, immovable, all-knowing, equally empowering as dangerous, summoned by lanes of chlorine and water.

I rely on his presence; I don't know who I am in the water without it.

As I approach the wall, my face in the pool, the shining square tiles on the floor become beacons among the dark stretched shadows of the rope lanes.

Mark's voice becomes a line I follow, he signals my tumble turn.

Feet flat on the wall, knees bent and push away . . .

Boys can crave attention, love, care from more than one man, the same way we can crave more than one friend, and Mark is part of the tenderly chosen family, one voice of many in my head.

Truthfully, I still struggle to find a grounding voice inside me, one that keeps me afloat. I've spent years in different kinds of therapies that attempt to tune you in to the narrative of how you experience yourself, your life; therapies that try to steer your story and soften the critic inside you, to understand that the language you use on yourself is a choice, a habit, that you must try not to get too stuck back and forth between the walls of trauma, that you have to get out of your lane.

It's Mark's voice that pushes me, one I will use when teaching my son to swim, a gentle rhythm, a pace, a style, a place along the lanes. That's what I crave when swimming, the meditation-like state, the loosening, lightening entering of a blue blurry underwater world of coordinated arms, legs, and breaths.

The lane shrinks you, confines your focus, and organizes your attention in a way that makes everything measurable. Your laps and strokes are easily self-managed and the clocks ticking on the walls offer an accurate portrayal of your speed and pace.

Swimming is cathartic too. In ancient Greece, catharsis was a physical practice, the original meaning being to "cleanse, purge"—you wake up every day with particular sorrows and struggles and each day you connect with them, get in the water and exorcize them.

If we're successful, we integrate our struggles into our lives rather than numb ourselves to them.

So I've kept swimming, and kept swimming, because the brain and heart are 73 percent water, and the brain constantly renews itself unless it is traumatized, when it is kept in the same murky pool, back-and-forthing.

The water in my lane is my past, my DNA, my memory (inherited and acquired), my father and everything he did, said, gave, and lost, his council home, his family. The water is the Victorian house my mother squatted in, my father's drinking, my sister's disappearances, the boy who stabbed me, the boy who loved me, the boy I was afraid of, the boy who was afraid of me, the boy calling me ugly, my nose too wide, head too square, my father calling me black, the black boy calling me white, the confusion distilling into self-hatred, the things I couldn't hear when they were said aloud, the things I didn't understand when they were written down. The water is everything I couldn't say, the codes spoken in streets, classrooms, behind the doors of head teachers' offices; my language couldn't cope with the visceral-ness, the feeling, the forced numbness. The water is everything I couldn't sit down and straighten out until now; this way I am able to tell the story the way I felt it, instead of the way I was told it. The power is in knowing the story I needed to hear, the story I needed to tell, but what is the story I need? Is it the same as the story I'm telling?

When it comes to water, it doesn't matter; it floats, lightens, and I move my body in sync despite it, because of it, because of it.

6

Blanche Nevile Deaf School

Camden Market was a bustling crowd of spiky-haired punks in metal-studded jackets, men in trench coats carrying guitars under their arms with cigarettes hanging out the side of their mouths, Goth women in black baggy jeans and powdered pale white faces, skinny shriveled-up bodies that shuffled through the crowds barging into shoulders and having you check your pockets as they passed. The Rastas (many of them cousins) blasting music by the canal through sound systems, selling cassette tapes, vinyl records, and red, green, and gold bracelets, necklaces and flags with the Lion of Judah wearing a gold crown beside posters of Haile Selassie and Marcus Garvey. Then, the man with the dark shades selling boxes of Baoding balls with yin and yang symbols painted on them as smoke from Chinese incense sticks wafted upward, someone nearby playing flute music, someone else pumping techno, the English woman with an eye patch and two dogs with three legs selling Moroccan carpets, next to the short Italian woman with jet-black curly hair and bright red lipstick selling silver rings, next to the black man with a stubble beard in a flat cap selling brown leather belts and black leather jackets. Everyone was a story, characters from a Steinbeck novel or a Bob Dylan song. It is true that Bob Dylan himself passed my mother's jewelry stall in 1995, wearing a black top hat, holding a black-and-white cane. Some call the late eighties, early nineties the peak cultural time of Camden Market and evoke nostalgia for those noncorporate, edgier times; there was always tension and mystery amid the vibrant randomness of market chaos. I loved it and blended in as a child of that market. I wore baggy T-shirts, sports tracksuit bottoms, and trainers, all of which often had holes in them by the end of the day from climbing on the railings near the Safeway car park behind the market, or playing football with a coked-up crusty punk who decided to boot my ball into a tree, or the shirtless Irish kids who ran away with the ball to have me chase them through the crowds down a street where their older brothers were waiting with knuckle-dusters and sticks.

If I worked at my mum's stall both weekend days, I could afford to buy myself a CD from Tony.

Tony was a short and intensely muscular black man with a tightly groomed goatee and biceps that almost burst out of his tight white T-shirts. If it was cold he wore a woolly scarf and beanie hat but his arms remained exposed as if the muscle itself had heat insulation.

He stood behind the crates of records and CDs bouncing along to whatever music he pressed play on.

"Yes, young star! What you after?"

Barely hearing him over his pumping music I pointed at his hip-hop and rap crate. Tony nodded as I picked out a CD with a silver case that said:

FLIPMODE SQUAD

I opened the case to look inside the jacket. I saw five black people, each posing in baggy tracksuits, a tall, slender dreadlocked black man stood in the center. I bought the album based on that picture—there was something about the attitude, the stance, the look I had wanted to share, be part of. My dad had taken me to Brick Lane the week before to buy a secondhand CD player that also had a tape deck I could record on. I got home and played Flipmode Squad the whole week, then the following week.

Tony slid a CD across his crates. "You bought Flipmode last week so you'll like this." The album cover was of a hazy explosion, a dark desolation; at the top it read "Busta Rhymes Extinction Level Event"—the dreads man from Flipmode Squad had a solo album, his name was Busta Rhymes.

Busta's wild energy and lyrical elasticity were barely contained by my cheap speakers, but I was enthused, bopping my head in a complete trance, taken in a major way by Busta's Jamaican inflections. I kept my hearing aids out to listen to him.

He was a fusion of a hip-hop and ragga artist; Dad had played many ragga artists like Barrington Levy, Beenie Man, Bounty Killer, Sister Nancy to me, but I found a deeper connection with Busta Rhymes because he combined his Jamaican-ness with his New York City–ness to create this eclectic bombastic vocal and lyrical dexterity; creativity oozed, huffed, puffed from his bravado, he projected an athleticism with his style. I wanted to know everything about this man, who evoked the sensibility of the Jamaican reggae and ragga artists that brought so much of my father's life and island to life.

Friends had noticed my Busta Rhymes obsession and the ones that knew his music, like Greg, my sister's boyfriend, and some of the boys I played football with on the weekend, started calling me "Bus-a-bus" (which punned my surname Antrobus). I then noticed multiple puns at play with the Busta name: Bust-a-rhyme, as in speak or present your words and make them rhyme and make sense.

At my dad's flat he got cable TV to lure me around to his place more often. He started recording music videos from the stations The Box and MTV Base, which played hip-hop and R&B. As I sat in front of a steaming plate of pork chops, fried onions, yam, and green banana, my dad played the music video for "What's It Gonna Be?!" featuring Janet Jackson, which was my first time seeing moving images of Busta Rhymes—every bit as cartoony and large as his vocals, my dad, rubbing the patch of beard below his lip, chuckled the whole way through. My father, noting the name, said he might be referring to Alexander Bustamante, the Jamaican labor leader on the island in the year in the 1970s when Busta Rhymes (real name, Trevor George Smith, Jr.) was born.

Crouched on the floor in my bedroom, I recorded my DIY radio shows onto cassette tapes as my two alter egos, DJ Check and DJ Check Mate. Busta Rhymes became my main imaginary guest as an uncontainable chaotic screaming presence who would grunt and gnash and wail like the *Looney Tunes* Tasmanian Devil.

I would individually record Busta Rhymes ad-libs and snippets of his vocals that he often performed alongside his hype man, Spliff Star, incorporating those sounds into the interview so I wouldn't have to impersonate him.

Me: Busta Rhymes, welcome to the studio with DJ Check!

Busta Rhymes: *GOT YOU ALL IN CHECK!*

Me: Glad to have you here. Now, you have a new song?

Busta Rhymes: *WHOO HA WHOO HA!*

Schools in Hackney were notoriously bad at the time. Hackney Downs boys' school had closed down in 1995 after multiple teachers were stabbed and one teacher died. As well as that, Hackney deaf education was underfunded, despite it being the borough with the first deaf school in England, a legacy that still isn't well managed or properly claimed by Hackney Council.

Traditionally, deaf children in London were sent to Mary Hare, Laycock, Oak Lodge, or Frank Barnes, but my mother wasn't convinced these schools suited me; there was either too much separation between the deaf and hearing students or too much focus on deafness and sign language. I needed a balance of both. Mainstream schools at most offered me in-class notetakers, but this seemed too passive. I needed engagement from teachers of the deaf.

At one school I visited with my first teacher of the deaf, Penny (who my mother had met after reaching out to Hackney Council for advice), and my mother, I was shown the assembly hall, which had microphones throughout the room to boost and amplify the voices in the space. Penny left, shaking her head. The children weren't allowed to sign; instead they used speech therapy and hearing aids, meaning that students weren't being supported in coming to terms with their deafness but in masking it to blend into a hearing world.

After deciding against schools within my catchment area, Penny had her mind on one school. Blanche Nevile. It was seven miles from Hackney—two bus journeys and a short walk, which meant one hour twenty minutes to school each way every day. I was offered a seat on a school bus, which would pick me up at 7:20 A.M. and get me to school for 8:40, registration at 8:45. I trusted Penny and agreed to attend the school.

Blanche Nevile was the name of the deaf school attached to Fortismere, the mainstream school. I had to register in both schools, in the morning in Blanche Nevile, in the afternoon, Fortismere, compounding this sense of myself as simultaneously belonging in two registers.

I was in the school for a year when I noticed that the Fortismere register kept forgetting me. My name kept disappearing from class lists: a mistake, of course—I had fallen through some crack, slipped between lists—but every time I sat in those mainstream classrooms without my name being called I felt invisible.

The first time I walked into Blanche Nevile deaf school the room was lit with bright strobes of fluorescent lights, the kind that feel clinical. I sat at one small square table next to another boy called Sam with brown hair and two large hearing aids, bigger than mine. We said nothing.

Three boys barged into the room, their voices wailing, an unrestrained screeching that broke through all the barriers of my socialized sound etiquette that was shushed into me by my hearing parents. Their arms freely flailing, and hands gesturing, they made a noise that was, to me, hoarse, stark, and crude. The attention they drew made me flinch. One of the boys turned to me and, with his hands, gestured and spoke in a way that sounded distorted, tuned out. He had a palm out so it faced his chest, with his other hand he raised four fingers from behind his fenced palm, which to me looked like toast popping out of a toaster.

"Toast?" I asked, thinking he was asking me what I had for breakfast.

The boy scrunched up his face, confused, then rapped his forehead with his knuckles.

"Mad, mad," he said and spun, crashed, and twirled his body to the back of the class.

A teacher, Miss Mukassa, a black woman with short, twisted dreads, strolled in, held the register, and calmly called out the names while another teacher (a woman whose name I've forgotten) stood beside her and gestured with her face and arms. I did everything I could to avoid eye contact with the gesturing woman, to pretend she was a void. I was self-conscious, unable to connect. When my name was called, I kept my whole body still as a satellite, eyes, ears, and all my hidden antennae silently picking up signals. This made me look strange to many of the other students, who interpreted it as arrogance or eccentricity.

I felt embarrassed in that room; the chairs were hard, the light overbearing, the walls quietly glaring. It was as if I was starting language all over again, being in a space where none of Renata's lessons could keep me afloat. I had never seen sign language before, so to me it just looked like a hyperactive drama performance and I didn't want to participate.

I was first taught to sign in a small classroom with one window in constant shade. Whatever weeds and vines reached the glass starkly stared. I remember it as an atmosphere of quiet shame, a world away from Renata's room. My BSL teacher, a woman with long grayish-blond hair, was nonverbal and only spoke in sign. When she wanted the attention of the class she banged on the table and made a loud wailing noise. She stood behind a poster of the alphabet, showing us the sign for each letter. By the end of the term, whoever's fingers spelled the BSL alphabet the fastest would be given a merit. Then by the next term, whoever could finger-spell a given word the fastest would win more merits. If you got enough merits you got a letter home that acknowledged your excellence.

Her teaching was effective. I learned the BSL alphabet quickly and it was from her that I found out that the boy on the first day was signing the word "new" to me and not "toast." I shared that story with her, which she laughed at and gave me a sign name, "Toast Boy."

Once I had learned the BSL alphabet I started using it to befriend some of the nonverbal, profoundly deaf students. But sign language still felt like something I had to hide from the hearing world, sensing the stigma and the ridicule it invited. I noticed some of the Fortismere students laughing and mocking a Blanche Nevile student who they saw signing as they walked to class. It made me wish that everyone learned BSL, that it could blend into the culture and not just be for the hundred or so kids packed in the deaf school.

Most of my academic lessons took place in Fortismere. When I started socializing there, making my friends (and enemies), some of them saw me use sign and asked why I was doing "that spastic thing" and it immediately shut me down. I stopped using sign when outside Blanche Nevile and eventually I stopped using sign altogether. I realized I had to pick a side, deaf or hearing. I quickly chose hearing; they were the majority, and the world I had more language for.

When I was twelve my sign name in Blanche Nevile changed from "Toast Boy" to the BSL letter "R" and the sign for "cap" because all the Blanche Nevile students noticed I started covering my ears, growing my hair long, and wearing hats, hoods, anything that hid my hearing aids. I was embarrassed, ashamed of my deaf parts, and I had to cover them up to integrate into the hearing world.

London in the late 1990s was embodied by a poster of the black British R&B star Mark Morrison that my close friend Adam (whose mother also worked at the markets) had put up in his bedroom. A black man with trimmed short, gelled, shiny hair wearing wide-framed dark shades, a gold chain, a black-and-yellow puffer jacket, grinning with a single gold tooth; in his pocket a pair of handcuffs—this was the Mack. He projected a suave toughness, the way we boys ought to hold ourselves. Adam and I would dress up as Morrison (he would lend me his clothes) while miming his hit "Return of the Mack" in his mother's mirror. The London I was growing up in was full of danger and all of it had to be navigated. The boys kicking footballs against the sides of the houses were bored and angry, the sex workers standing outside telephone boxes on the corner were cold and desperate, the men holding beer bottles and shouting on the park benches were often hungry and homeless. Mark Morrison seemed to be the template, to project enough danger to keep yourself safe. Unfortunately for me, I couldn't project that suave, tough, masculine image. Even the clothes I borrowed from Adam never fit properly and, yes, I removed my hearing aids whenever I sang "Return of the Mack" in the mirror.

I filled my school holidays with trips to sports centers to play indoor football and swimming pool leisure centers to meet girls. Sometimes girls would seem to like me at first, meeting in the pool, but after seeing the way I dressed—baggy T-shirts and fake Adidas tracksuit bottoms with holes in them—they gave me a fake number and ran away.

At Fortismere and Blanche Nevile there were many more ethnicities and cultures to mix with and suddenly asserting my identity within the school was essential for survival. In Fortismere, my status and identity were challenged. There was no uniform, everything I wore was baggy: Fubu shirts, Sean John jeans, and tracksuits. On my way to a class one day an older boy barged into me.

"Fassy," he said. "You think you're black." He was white. In order to assert my blackness, my position, it wasn't enough to present Busta Rhymes, to wear baggy clothes, "buss sags" as it was called. I had to actually "look black."

Neither of my parents seemed to anticipate that I would have to define and defend my blackness to everyone outside my family, which was also true of my deafness. In my mind I was figuring out how to be socially safe, loved by my family, and respected by my peers. I had internalized an idea that asserting my blackness would provide love, as would hiding my deafness. I had many black people who I considered "worthy of love" to put on my bedroom wall, but no deaf ones. When the boy said *you think you're black,* he may as well have said *you're unlovable to everyone you care about.*

There's a photo of my father with five of his brothers all standing shoulder to shoulder in a flat somewhere in England, all smiling with their teeth except my father, with a slighter, closed-mouth smile. His brothers' complexions vary from olive-skinned with curly clouds of hair and a thick mustache that made them look Mexican, to the clean-shaven light caramel complexion with short wavy hair that looked Cuban. Some had straighter hair than others and my father was the least ambiguously black, with his wide nose, afro, and dark skin, but all of them came from the same parents, an ancestry thought to be a mix of Arawak Indian, West African, and Scottish, perceived as "coolies" or "Taínos" or "blacks" in Jamaica and flattened into "West Indians" in England. The spectrum of my father and his brothers' complexions and hair textures carried their mix of history and meant that my father could look at my olive complexion and straighter hair and still see a boy as smoothly black as him. But the sophistication that was required to define me as black was not applied to defining me as deaf. The framework wasn't there: Deafness had no spectrum, no family ties, no history, no culture or language, remember? The only word my father gave it was "limited."

In geography I was one of two Blanche Nevile students in the Fortismere class. The other was Sam. We were thirteen and fourteen. It was the only class we had together without a support teacher. I didn't understand why it was decided we wouldn't need support in geography; perhaps there was a staff shortage and geography wasn't a core subject like English and math.

Sam and I wrote notes to each other throughout the lesson, helping each other if something was missed or needed clarification.

I developed a crush on a girl in the class and suddenly felt embarrassed that she could see Sam and me writing notes, needing support.

It was that week I stepped late into class, no hat and a new trim, no hair to cover my ears. I had taken my hearing aids out and announced a lie to the class:

"I don't need hearing aids anymore."

Everyone (except Sam) erupted in applause as if I'd won a new ranking in the order of things, while Sam remained where he was and slowly sank below his desk.

As I sat, Sam grabbed my geography book and wrote:

How come you don't wear hearing aids anymore?

I wrote back:

I just don't need them.

The geography teacher, Mr. Boyd, took no special interest in my needs and the lack of hearing aids in my ears. This was my idea of liberation; even if it meant I was missing parts of the lessons it was more important for me to superficially blend in with hearing people.

If I were to find my old, creased green geography books and look for all the words, anything that had passed between Sam and me, all I would find are the unfinished diagrams of water cycles, the weather between abandoned friends.

Miss Willis was still teaching in Blanche Nevile when I returned nearly two decades later for a residency. She greeted me with pride and excitement when I stepped into her classroom again. The school was in a different building now, no longer hidden in the bushes; it was out in the open, announcing itself along the footpath of Fortismere North Wing. Miss Willis introduced me to her class of seven students, who sat around square tables, students who signed, spoke. Miss Willis filled me in on what she knew of my old classmates, who was doing well and who was struggling.

Miss Willis selected four students with relatively decent English literacy skills. Most of the profoundly deaf Blanche Nevile students had low English literacy due to reasons sometimes outside of deafness, such as other neurodivergent needs. I realized that if I was a teenager today, I would likely be mainstreamed. I would not be deaf or disabled enough to be at Blanche Nevile now: For most of the students, deafness was just one of several disabilities.

The four students I had were all cochlear implanted—meaning they had their hearing devices surgically placed within their ears. They signed, spoke, and were lip-readers who wrote fairly fluently. They were assertive, confident, forthcoming in wanting to contribute to the lessons, asking questions (in both BSL and English). It was inspiring for me to see integrated deaf young people who were able to thrive in ways that I struggled to at their age. There's an old idea that deaf people struggle with abstraction: How can a sign truly convey the meaning of ideas that can't be touched or shaped? Words like religion, enlightenment, divine?

In 1742, an eccentric French teacher of the deaf, Abbé Roch-Ambroise Sicard, staged public performances with his most articulate and gifted deaf students for the general (hearing) public with the aim of showcasing the results of his own teaching practices. He was fame-hungry and selling himself as the most celebrated teacher of the deaf in France. These performances grew so popular there were special private shows for the pope, the archbishop of Paris, and other high-ranking figures.

Each performance lasted around four hours as the deaf students of Sicard were brought onto the stage to exhibit their language and comprehension skills in written French and French Sign Language. A blackboard was placed on the stage to prove students could write French sentences as well as sign them. Sicard would ask his audience of three hundred spectators for "the day's *Gazette*" newspaper. Articles from the paper would be signed for the audience by the students, then written in French on the blackboard. Sicard asked questions, signaling out the abstract words like government, arrondissement, department and instructing the students to define them in writing and sign. The audience was sold at this point, but Sicard went further by inviting questions from the audience.

Massieu, one of the students, was asked, "What is God?"

Massieu wrote: "The Necessary Being, the sun of eternity, the mechanist of nature, the eye of justice, the watchmaker of the universe, the soul of the universe."

Massieu's use of metaphor and imagery proved the sophistication of his thinking and, to the hearing people gathered, the humanity of the deaf.

In classrooms, I admit, it can sometimes be a challenge to explain figurative language to the Deaf, but just as with any language, if you're skilled and confident in sign, you find creative ways to express it. Visual vernacular, international sign language, regional signs all contribute to the Deaf vocabulary. For years, my main use of sign has been SSE (Sign Supported English), which is not its own language but an aid to English speech, unlike BSL, which is a five-hundred-year-old language with its own syntax and grammar structure. In poetry, there is a sign language called Signart, which is separate from spoken and written language poetry. "Written poetry is for the hearing," says Deaf BSL poet John Wilson. "We [the Deaf] have our own poetry."

In 1957, the Deaf Welsh poet Dorothy Miles, known as "Dot" to her close friends, enrolled in Gallaudet University in Washington, DC.

Miles won a scholarship to leave her home in the UK and study psychology at the university. She was twenty-six with a background in theater, already an enthusiast of Shakespeare and writing her own poems and plays from a young age.

By 1958 the on-campus literary magazine began publishing her poems. Miles's early poems took nature as their theme, shying away from direct biographical details. But like Granville Redmond's landscape paintings, her depiction of nature mirrors the emotions of the author.

A poem titled "Fragments," published in 1959, begins:

> *A sunlit moor and a shifting, drifting pattern of cloud / beyond / A lonely farm, with a solemn column of ducks on a minute / pond / These are the things that come rising out of the mists where old memories lie / to catch the heart, with an aching, shaking longing for days gone by.*

This early pastoral poem in English has foundational similarities in tone and image to a much later poem of Miles's, not in English but BSL, "Cloud Magic." You can watch Miles perform it on YouTube. Her BSL signs are fluid and dramatic, shaping the clouds in the air and representing the shock of them with a quick opening of her palms above her head, as if the clouds are inspiring excitement, but also danger and mystery. There are no humans in this poem, only animals; she signs "sheep," "bull," "pigs," she signs and shapes each of their facial expressions as they notice the clouds and transcend into the sky, all of them noticing birds among the magic clouds, watching them wistfully, bringing a sense of yearning for flight to the earthbound animals toward the end, a tone also rendered in "Fragments" with the "shaking, aching" verbs she blends into signs.

Miles had both a hearing and Deaf identity; though she was profoundly deafened in childhood she retained her speech. Miles acquired spoken English before her deafness and signed BSL shortly afterward. She learned ASL (American Sign Language) at Gallaudet and eventually integrated all her signed, spoken, and written languages into her poetry. She referred to her early poems as "just verse," whereas her poems in her 1976 collection *Gestures* experimented with what she called "blending or interlinking." *Gestures* was accompanied with footage of Miles performing poems in BSL, standard English, and a mix of sign and English or just sign.

Miles was one of the most skillfully rounded Deaf poets in the UK in her time, yet despite her range of written English and sign poems, many people outside of the Deaf world have not come across her. What inspires me about her is that she refused to compartmentalize herself or her language into singular assimilating forms; her integrity and commitment to the hybridity of her deaf sensibilities remain a guiding light.

When Sicard was exhibiting his deaf students, Massieu was often asked by the audience to explain music. Massieu described music as "an agreeable sensation excited by the voice or the sound of instruments." The idea that the deaf do not have music is a myth that won't die. Many of the mainstream stories of deafness coming out of Hollywood, like the films *Sound of Metal* and *CODA,* center around the idea of music as a source of conflict for the deaf, which is, at worst, a harmful stereotype that excludes the joy of music from the deaf.

Deaf percussionist Dame Evelyn Glennie points out that "most deaf people do not live in a world of silence." Most people, hearing or deaf, have some relationship with sound and music. Any conversation about deaf people that doesn't honor this complexity reduces the rich life of music that many deaf people enjoy.

My particular experience of music is that I don't hear softer, higher sounds; details in the percussion like bells, whistles, bird sounds, and softly spoken voices are lost to me. I didn't listen to much instrumental music growing up. I needed words and I needed the voice delivering those words to have bass, depth, presence, something that carried their meaning to my ears over the beat.

I fell in love with Tupac's voice in part for the way he stretched out his end and internal rhymes; he made music out of the parts of speech I struggle with most; he had a clarity to his flow that was smooth, intricate but unforced, and, to my ear, pitch-perfect. My sister once noted that I listen to a lot more music by men than women, and my deafness is part of that because I tend to resonate more with deeper voices.

Later, Leonard Cohen, Tracy Chapman, Miriam Makeba, and Nina Simone would become some of my most listened to artists. All have striking, clear, lyrical, and emotional voices, voices that lean me closer to them but also want me to hear their words. Everything feels weighed, considered. Any extra work they put on my ear is worth it and they rarely let me down.

My mother played Leonard Cohen's "One of Us Cannot Be Wrong" on the cassette player in her bedroom. I could barely tell if the deep voice was speaking or singing but I registered a profound yearning in it. I didn't wear my hearing aids at home unless I really wanted to hear something with full intention—his voice had me putting them in, turning them up. With my hearing aids in, the vocals were clear and forward-facing over the gentle guitar melody, the presence of the voice carrying the lyrics was so full and pronounced. I asked who it was and if I could listen to more.

My mum seemed surprised, but she showed me a selection of her CDs—a band called Traffic, John Lennon, George Harrison, Joe Cocker, white musicians. Noting this relieved me slightly because Mum blaring roots reggae in her Mini Metro when picking me up somewhere would turn heads, attracting attention and inviting scrutiny. Regardless, I kept Cohen a secret, recognizing that I had no peers around who would resonate with Cohen's soft, sincere sound, that it would be understood as "white."

At my dad's council flat in Dalston, where the living room was also a bedroom—a double bed in the corner, the TV facing the bed—was his sound system. One large hazelwood box speaker that stood up to my waist, and behind that was a curtained wide window. On the inside ledge he grew marijuana in little brown plant pots. On the wall at the side of his bed was a Jamaican flag and a portrait of my face taken from my last photo day in primary school. When it was taken, the photographer had repeatedly asked me to smile, to show teeth to *CHHHEEEEESSSEE,* but all I would give was the shy smirk that looked out from my father's wall for years.

I was sitting on the chair next to his bed, he was lying down with a spliff between his fingers, when I asked him if he'd heard of Leonard Cohen. "I prefer Dylan," he said, getting up to run his fingers through a box of cassette tapes. "I thought he was an old black man like Paul Robeson when I first heard it on the radio," he said as he recited the opening verse of "Blowin' in the Wind."

The air in my dad's flat was pungent; the strong tobacco and weed smoke clung to my clothes and hair. When he found the tape, Dylan's voice pulsed through the speaker; like Cohen, the vocals front and center, everything tuned toward the words. "I couldn't believe that was sung by some white Jewish kid." I nodded. I went home to tune in to hip-hop and R&B stations, my finger on the button ready to record anything that sounded like a groove, a hard beat, a mean flow, something I could project outward, a black sound I could be seen and heard with.

7

Deaf Anger

I can't recall how it started but I was in my mother's kitchen, chest-to-chest with my father, wide unblinking eye to wide unblinking eye. There was alcohol on his breath, tobacco smell in his beard and coat. "You think you bad?" he snarled, then turned his back and shot out the door. He picked up two bricks from my mother's garden and came back and stood with his nose almost touching mine. "You think you bad?" he said, louder. "Fuck you!" I said, and that was the first time I'd said that to his face. Then there was nothing left to say or do but hit him, but I saw him hesitate. We both hesitated.

I'd had dreams of buildings collapsing when he shouted; dreams of standing on a sinking ship, water rushing onto the deck and my drunk father both captain and the iceberg; dreams of my drunk father under a bridge like the troll in "Three Billy Goats Gruff." My father drunk seemed ruthlessly indestructible—

but this slight drop of his eyes, this evidence of a second thought that has me looking into my memory: The man is in the ground and still stands there with one momentary doubt that I never knew he was capable of. Does it mean he didn't really want it to come to this, this aggression, this threat of violence? And yet, what else was available for us? My drunk fuming father with a brick in each hand showed me one gesture of doubt, of things not being as he wanted them. My father wasn't muscled, he was slender. I knew he could throw a punch, because I still have two bald patches on the back of my head from where he swung at me with his ring finger after he caught me jumping on his bed as a child.

My mother ran into the kitchen and immediately jumped between us. My father dropped the bricks and they crashed onto the hardwood kitchen floor with a loud indoor thump that permanently dented and scratched it and would mean my mother would always cover that part with a thick red-and-black rug. Then my father turned his back and marched away.

My mother signed me up for anger management classes. I refused to go at first, but then she started driving me to the sessions. She sat in the room with me, explained to the therapist that I had been violent at home, that I had punched holes in the walls and smashed windows, that I frightened her, made her feel like shit, that my father was also abusive toward her and that I was probably getting it from him. I sat in the chair getting angrier and angrier. All my mother's stories felt less like someone trying to have an open conversation and more like an attack, an accusation, and the fury that was erupting in my teenage brain felt wrong, a source of my own shame. I don't remember anything being said about my deafness; I didn't have hearing aids in during the sessions, I kept them in my pocket and stared at the therapist, a black woman with long plaits and a friendly moon-shaped face. She had a pronounced east London accent that was clear in a quiet room.

It was mainly my mother doing the venting in those sessions anyway; she needed therapy as much as I did. She was a survivor of domestic abuse and the English era of postwar rationing. J.K. and Barbara would've done their best, but still passed on some of their own traumas to my mother and my mother to me.

The counselor, looking only at me, said to breathe deeper when I felt myself getting angry, to count from one to ten, visualize a calm beach with bright blue water, hear the waves and keep breathing.

Anger was something I instinctively knew not to show too publicly because it welcomed more conflict and scrutiny, leaving you more vulnerable.

I internalized some of this growing up with an alcoholic father. Publicly, people thought of my father as a charming, laid-back, easygoing "irie-vibe" Rastaman, but when he was drunk, he was volatile, violent, and belligerent. He beat me, and he beat my mother while shouting something incoherent about "white devils." Because his violence only occurred when he was drunk and behind closed doors, it signaled something to me about privatizing rage, holding it in for only those closest to bear it.

After my father's drunken rages he would black out and wake slumped on the sofa, having no memory of his destruction. Sometimes he'd see the glass from the milk bottles he'd smashed on our doorstep, stare at the scattered shards completely puzzled and ask, *Who did that?* It was such a routine that I didn't bother putting my hearing aids in when he was hungover. I knew all his lines. No one witnessed my father's fury except the walls, the doorsteps, and the faces of his family.

"I never quite knew how to deal with situations before they happened," said twenty-one-year-old deaf boxer Reece Cattermole after winning his first professional fight in York Hall in Bethnal Green in 2018, the same venue where I started swimming. Like me, Reece Cattermole is a mixed black man grown up in British society with a history of anger. He, like me, started anger management counseling as a teenager.

"Boxing helped me learn how different people communicate." Cattermole began boxing at eleven and was already in anger management to cope with the stress his deafness was causing him. He doesn't sign, he relies on lip-reading. The language of the face. In the ring, Cattermole's gaze is a fierce, unflinching focus, which he says his deafness helped him harness. "I might still hear background noise," he says, "but everything else is completely shut out."

Cattermole leans into his deafness and has created a fighter that is informed by it. Rather than a reason to shrink himself and avoid conflict as if it were inevitable, he has found a way to manage and channel his deafness into the sporting body. "Boxing takes your mind off a lot of things," he says. "Whatever you personally feel—anger, confusion, excitement—you can take it out on a bag without feeling any guilt."

Audiologists told Cattermole that he has a regenerative gene that means his hearing will progressively worsen; by forty he's expected to be profoundly deaf. He is the first deaf British boxer to be given a license since the 1970s.

I was fourteen in 2001 when my father bought me a punching bag. I had no technique and sprained my wrist after taking too hard a swing at it. After I healed, I was taken to a boxing club in north London to learn how to throw a punch. At the club a boy I knew from the estate was sparring in the ring. Because we were friendly with each other he invited me into the ring to spar with him. I took my hearing aids out and put on a red headguard. What I thought was going to be an easy training session ended with him knocking me flat onto the mat. I never went back.

Reece Cattermole stands outside of a brick wall after his debut professional fight, one side of his face purple and swollen. Stripes of bruising line his forehead and the interviewer points it out: "You got quite a few bruises." But Cattermole is quick to cut in. "I mean, obviously he did catch me, he is quite a good fighter . . . but you know"—he shrugs—"it's a learning process, you're always learning different things from different people." In all of Cattermole's interviews he uses this kind of language, the mode of the student, the learner, the eager wide-eyed scholar undertaking an apprenticeship in his passion.

As well as learning from his opponents, Cattermole's deafness means he also has to learn from referees. Referees have their own style of overseeing matches, their own pitched voices and speed and way of moving around the ring that Cattermole has to rely on. From outside the ring spectators may not notice how verbal and physical the referee is with the fight they are in charge of—*Break! Stop boxing!*—and they have to throw their own bodies between the boxers if a punch is thrown after the bell. Cattermole can't hear the bell so relies on the referee's physical presence more than any other professional boxer.

What moves me about Cattermole is that he fights on his own terms within the existing structures of the sport. Monitoring the referee, the rule-keeper of the fight, he anticipates how the referee will act before he makes a move. "You can read their body language when they're going to break fighters," says Cattermole. "When you're in the sport a while you pick these things up; besides it's the referee's role to make the boxers aware [of the rules/the bell]."

Because Cattermole is trained and has developed a style and sense of self in the ring, something that ought to go against him becomes creative, a new maneuver; he's proficient, a professional, and his skill keeps him as safe as one can be within striking distance of a hook, jab, or body blow.

Standing by the boxing ring, hearing aid turned up, Cattermole is asked how he feels about being a deaf boxer. A microphone is brought to his mouth, he looks straight-faced and serious, says, "I don't think it's a problem."

Cattermole wasn't born deaf, but, like me, he needs hearing aids, he lip-reads; to some he could pass for hearing, but that's not what he is. Just hearing and seeing him assert who he is with such (brutal) grace and integrity is inspiring, an embodied story that everyone (deaf, hearing, both) needs to see.

Tyrone Givans was in Blanche Nevile with me, a tall, handsome black boy with blue hearing aids who dyed his high-top bronze and wore hazel-colored contact lenses. He'd dance and sing, sign and speak to everyone, deaf or hearing. I remember seeing him through my classroom window running across the football pitch, the tick of his Nike trainers glowing as if affirming him, a chosen one. He was chased by a group of girls as if he was already a star. His laugh stretched his face out but I couldn't hear the sound (or is that my memory now?). If there's an end-of-school yearbook with Tyrone's face in it, it predicts him as "most likely to become famous." He was a rapper and a poet, writing in notebooks, dreaming of stardom.

Once, I saw Tyrone in a fistfight with another boy, a taller boy who was trained in kickboxing. Each of the punches connected, each blow Tyrone took without stumbling. It was as good as any professional fight: Neither boy won, so equally matched that both walked away cut, bruised, exhausted, but with respect and integrity attached to their names for the rest of their school years.

But after Tyrone left school, things slowly fell apart for him. Little of his glory and confidence seemed to translate in the world outside the school gates. He became isolated, losing contact with most of his friends in the deaf world. He worked jobs in supermarkets, leisure centers, and trained as an aerobics instructor, but he struggled to assimilate into the hearing world, staying at home and drinking until those jobs fell away from him.

Without a stable livelihood he developed alcoholism, his relationship with his girlfriend became volatile, and soon he ended up in jail on domestic abuse charges.

Tyrone was arrested without his hearing aids, and although he pleaded for them, they were not returned to him. He sat in his cell and sank deeper and deeper into isolation without his hearing aids to help him. There was a failure around his file, two different spellings of his name in the system, a mess and a mistake, which meant that the file that was pulled up when Tyrone was pleading for his hearing aids did not confirm that he was deaf.

Tyrone asked the prison staff for help, said that his mental health was suffering, but the prison counselor dismissed him with a prescription for alcohol withdrawal and antidepressants. The counselor said he didn't really need hearing aids because he seemed to communicate fine without them. This is a textbook example of audism, a term coined by Dr. Tom Humphries in 1975 at Gallaudet University. Its meaning describes the infrastructural oppression and discrimination against Deaf people who use sign language and Deaf culture.

Within days of this report, Tyrone went back to his cell and hanged himself. Miss Willis was at his funeral, wordless, standing in the pews with her hand over her mouth as the coffin was carried into the church.

Penny, the first teacher of the deaf I met at eleven, found me again after hearing me interviewed on BBC Radio 4 for Deaf Awareness Week. She messaged me online and we arranged to meet in her home the following week. I was excited and nervous, having spent so long thinking about and making sense of my childhood education. This was the woman who laid down the tracks, arranged in-class support, and got me accepted into Blanche Nevile deaf school—what might I owe her? What might she expect of me now?

I stood outside Penny's house. A London plane tree towered in front of it; its shadow swayed on the white-painted bricks. The street was coincidentally blocks away from the first school I taught poetry in more than a decade before, a mainstream Catholic school. In those classrooms I learned to incorporate my deafness into lessons, asking students to speak up when reading their poems to the class, reminding them I needed their voice projected. I played a game called "Volume Control," asking the students to stand in one long line. One end of the line represented high volume, the other end, low volume. I would ask the students to hold a humming note while I walked up and down the line like a human volume knob. The students hummed louder or quieter depending on where I stood along the line. I then stopped and stood at the frequency I needed their in-class voices to be: not too loud, not too quiet, right in the middle, between the loudest hum and the quietest.

I rang the bell and a woman with short-cropped hair and thin-rimmed black glasses emerged.

"Raymond, what a thing to see you, gosh!"

We embraced on the doorstep. I walked into the hallway, pausing by her bookshelves of Wordsworth complete editions. Penny tapped me on the shoulder so she could face me as she spoke and told me that "love" was the word Wordsworth used most in his poems, also "heart" and "eye."

I explained that what I most admired in Wordsworth was his championing of "common speech" in poems and that he argued against an elitist positioning of poetry.

Penny and I walked into her living room, a couch and two chairs facing each other. She knew how to lay out a room for a deaf person, a close face-to-face seating plan. Penny sat on the couch in front of the cushioned chair. "You'll see and hear me well from there." She looked into my face, taking me in; she last saw me when I was eleven years old.

"What a thing to see you, gosh!" she repeated.

She handed me an old copy of the *Hackney Gazette,* my local paper, from the 1990s. In it, there's a picture of the mayor of Hackney surrounded by waving and smiling children, three adults in spectacles (teachers of the deaf), and one woman in a black hat (the parent of a deaf child), and a ten-year-old Tyrone Givans in the bottom corner wearing a green-and-black coat and gray hearing aids, the only face with a grimace.

They are all standing by the plaque honoring the first deaf school in England, founded by Thomas Braidwood in 1783. I see Penny as I remembered her then, younger, with soft, friendly eyes. The headline, a pun that reads:

IT'S "SIGN" LANGUAGE—SITE OF FIRST DEAF SCHOOL MARKED WITH PLAQUE

I wanted to know what Penny thought about the complicated significance of Braidwood's school and its exclusivity—where would Tyrone or I come into this history?

"It meant something to have this heritage unhidden, to point at this site and say what began," said Penny, but the black boy crouching down in front of her in the photo distracted me. I put my finger on his face.

"That's Tyrone," I said and covered my mouth.

Penny had no idea what had happened to him. I told her what I remembered of Tyrone from school, his kindness and talent, his popularity and the fight he got into on the football field, how he had held his own against one of the hardest pupils in the hearing school, how that fight meant no one picked on any deaf kids for the rest of the year. I hated that I had to end the story at his funeral. Penny's face dropped.

"Yes, it's hard for deaf black boys, and I felt protective of you for that too." Penny got up from the sofa to make tea, and we didn't speak for a few minutes, needing to process what was said so far.

She returned to the sofa, placing two steaming mugs of tea on the table in front of us. "As a child in my care," said Penny, "you were part of a family unit. I remember your sister and mum and I remember hearing about your dad and understood that was an important relationship. I remember you must have been a child with good coping strategies because there was always a push to say you were all right, you were fine."

The same was said about Tyrone. We cope until we can't take the stress of trying to be understood anymore. The way we are seen and understood has to be explained to figures of authority; we are in danger if we can't do that. Tyrone and I, both being Caribbean British boys, citizens of the British state, were vulnerable to systemic discrimination. Black Caribbean British and mixed boys were more likely to be excluded from school than their white, African British, and mixed counterparts.

"I was interested in you as a mixed Jamaican child," said Penny. "I knew some of the challenges, there was a feeling I had to do more for you because of that, but we didn't develop the relationship well enough to explore that. That could've been helpful, but I guess you wouldn't have known how to articulate that for yourself, same way I wouldn't know how to write a poem."

Our mugs were empty. Hours had already whizzed by. I stood up to put my coat on, walking back past her bookshelves. I picked up one of the heavyset volumes of Wordsworth's complete works, flicked through for my favorite poem of his, and, not finding it, recited the opening line: "The world is too much with us," I said, "late and soon."

Penny and I stood at the door smiling at each other. What else to say with our words? I hope I said, "Thank you, Penny, you did more for me than you'll ever know," but I'm not sure I did. I think I was politely calm and mild-mannered but thinking through our shared history felt emotionally turbulent. I think I said, "You know, you were my first teacher of the deaf," and Penny said something about her first teacher of the deaf, a man who inspired her to pursue deaf education, how she had said to her first teacher of the deaf that she didn't understand why there was so much prejudice against the deaf, the denial of their education and language, the social shunning, the shaming of welfare, when any one of us could find ourselves deaf tomorrow. "My teacher laughed at that," said Penny, "and I never found out why he found it so funny."

A few days later, processing our conversation, I thought of all the nameless teachers who go above and beyond for their students, working unpaid overtime, writing letters of recommendation, noting their potential, selflessly rooting for and believing in them.

Of course, I thought too of Tyrone, that not all of Penny's

students made it, that you can only do so much, and then hope it's enough.

I sent Penny a text message, asking what she thought of her legacy. I was curious: How does one honor teachers for their care and guidance, a love, heart, and eye that got them through?

She texted back: "I just wanted the people I worked with, hearing or deaf, to be capable of forming good relationships, there isn't a better thing I could do in the world than help people have good relationships . . . it's as basic as that."

I'm visiting Gallaudet University, the only university in the world where all classes are designed specifically for the D/deaf. "Electric Relaxation" by A Tribe Called Quest is playing on the radio. At Gallaudet University Deaf poet Christopher Jon Heuer, a large man with the presence of a friendly bull, meets me. He notices my hearing aids instantly and asks if I sign ASL (American Sign Language). I tell him I sign basic BSL. "We won't understand each other, I'll type on my phone," he says. Should I tell him that isn't necessary because I'm hard of hearing rather than profoundly deaf and he has a deep bass voice? But he's already typing his name in the notes section of his phone and walking us toward the statue of Thomas Gallaudet. He types out the history of the campus, the significance of Edward and Thomas Gallaudet, then hands it to me. There's a slight wind blowing into my hearing aids, which muffles everything. Then I'm moved by Christopher's consideration for me. People usually assume my hearing is better than it actually is and I end up feeling a pressure to uphold that impression. Some people have told me I sometimes have a "nervous energy" but it's usually because those people have voices I struggle to hear, but with Christopher typing I don't have to make that extra effort to lip-read or fill in the blanks of our conversation. As he hands me his phone with all the information in text, I instantly feel a rare kind of relief.

Christopher guides us onto the campus and types, "Do you have these video booths in the UK?" He sits in the booth and explains how deaf people call an operator on the screen, then the conversation can be signed or captioned. He points at the buttons and waits for my eyes to meet his face and says, "This is how the deaf can speak to anyone."

I think of all the times I was nervous to call the bank or the cinema, knowing the operator wouldn't speak clearly or loud enough. I think of the black clunky rubber pads I had to put on the receiver so I could speak on the phone with my hearing aids in, how I would push the receiver so hard into the side of my head trying to hear the operator, the pads marking my skin and leaving my ears burning bright red.

I excuse myself, trying not to weep. I think of the stories head teachers in deaf schools had told me about some parents who were ashamed of their child's deafness, how they spoke like grieving parents, begging them to "make my child speak." Then I sob audibly, thinking of the stories I'd heard about the isolation some deaf elderly people experience, how long they have to wait to speak to a GP with an interpreter; tears stream down my face and I'm embarrassed.

Christopher asks if I'm okay. I'm not able to explain in the moment why I'm crying, why I'd never seen anything like this in a public setting before, but Christopher doesn't make a big deal out of my tears. He leads me to the bookshop and I'm standing in an aisle among books, mostly written by D/deaf authors, on teaching, learning sign, deaf literature, history, and poetry, and it hits me again, other memories of feeling alone in my condition, completely unaware there was a library of people who share a frequency with my experience, and, yes, as I write this now, I'm thinking again of Tyrone. What connected us, what failed us, what world could be made for us?

8

Johnnie Ray

America heard Johnnie Ray croon for the first time through the radio in the autumn of 1951 and no one tuned in like the misunderstood misfits did, the ones who felt strange and awkward in their complicated bodies. Ray's singing swung with so much feeling, was so alive and aligned with such pleading sorrow, that myths blossomed all around him.

Ray knew a thing or two about the public and private performance of the deaf body. A skinny, sensitive, bisexual deaf boy from the suburbs, he grew up to become the brief spotlit white face of Black American music.

At first they mistook his voice for a Black woman and music executives and critics alike grimaced, said that "she" lacked smoothness and precision in her phrasing. When they found out that Ray wasn't a Black woman, that he was a white deaf man from Dallas, Oregon, they changed their tune and dubbed him "The Prince of Wails."

Johnnie Ray had been touched by Black sound since he was a teenager. He first heard Billie Holiday and whatever wave hit him never left. But that wasn't the only thing that struck me when I first watched the grainy black-and-white footage of Ray crooning in the spotlight—it was also his unconcealable boxy hearing aid.

In 1948, before Ray's first performance in the Flame, the lavish liberal downtown venue in Detroit where he would be discovered, Ray was told, "The louder you sing, boy, the better," and, believe me, Ray brought his volume beyond the stage. He took his microphone from the stand and strolled into the audience, his boxy hearing aid device so heavily amplified that every ear must have felt the static and spit. The Flame presented the biggest Black names in music at the time, from Billie Holiday to Dinah Washington. It was the Midwest's leading live showcase for jazz, R&B, and Black variety artists. Patronized by both the Black working class and high-class white liberals, its five-hundred-seat capacity was reached nightly.

"Flame Show Bar" was spelled out in huge neon letters on either side of a diagonal corner marquee and entrance. Its interior was luxurious with a long bar and a sunken nightclub floor, and dozens of tables crowded in a semicircle around the stage. On each table there were gavel-like wooden knockers that audience members could beat to blare their approval of an act.

Despite the Flame announcing Black lineups, Ray was the exception—although some say he was so caked in makeup under the light that he often looked like a Black man or an Italian.

The visible presence of his hearing aid (which was perhaps another sign that Ray was "other" enough to be embraced on Black stages) meant he got away with not being on beat. His band helped him along. If Ray fell away from the tempo, they pumped their horns and drums louder and sometimes held back to wait for Ray to find himself again in the rhythm.

The singer LaVern Baker was in the audience that night and said that Ray's deafness meant "he could get away with murder," musically. But tonight Ray was a lanky, liberated androgynous-looking twenty-two-year-old. When he arrived at the climax of his performance, wailing lung-bursting blues at such high decibels that the whole stage vibrated below his feet, his sweat-soaked shirt displayed to the audience, his wide trembling arms, and his voice wild and flexed with such visceral inner energy that no ear or eye could hold together, no one moved, nothing except whatever released Ray from his stiff and awkward constraints was now bared and glowing in the spotlight.

Ray found himself onstage in the Flame Show Bar where his future manager and lover, Bill Franklin, sat in his pressed smooth blue suit and white shirt and saw a frail figure stand in the spotlight, snapping his large long, long fingers to a beat that hadn't begun.

You can't believe everything that went down in a smoky midnight downtown Detroit bar, but I can believe that everything hushed as Ray poured his whiskey-and-gin voice, I can believe that the air changed color as Ray crooned into the darkness. Later, Bill would say that Ray was never more himself than in his early days performing here, in "black and tan joints," where he was "a much wilder, bolder, much more secure performer."

Some music critics called Ray melodramatic on the stage; they hated how he held himself, how he pretended to faint, tumbling theatrically over the body of the piano; hated how he picked up his music stand and pounded it into the ground as if some colorful current had shot up in his suit and he'd imploded with it. Later in his career beyond the Flame Show Bar, his booking agents saw Ray's hearing aid as a hindrance, something that boxed him into a gimmicky novelty act, a "handicapped honky," a "vehicle for self-pity." But Ray soon proved his talent had staying power, life beyond the dimension of novelty or caricature, when he began consistently selling out acclaimed clubs across America and acquainting himself with adored Hollywood stars from Marlon Brando and Sammy Davis, Jr., to Marilyn Monroe and Fred Astaire. Before he started stepping onto more mainstream stages like New York's Copacabana, he would be forced to sing without his hearing aid, which led to stiffer performances. On those stages, Ray could barely hold himself in time, staying put between the piano and the drummer, relying on the vibration and eye contact with the band.

There was always cynicism about Ray being a deaf novelty act. A *New York Times* critic even said, "His performance is the anatomy of self-pity." But if you listen right, what comes out of his performance is the image of a man and a child, barely holding himself together. In the end nothing and nobody hurt or beat Ray up more than himself.

Jonny Whiteside wrote in his biography of Ray, *Cry,* that "popular music relies on gauging and defining an audience's self-image and desires, the unspoken urges that lie at the soul's core. By speaking to and gratifying the needs of its audience, pop music goes beyond entertainment to offer spiritual glamour." But there was nothing glamorous, spiritual, or liberating about Ray—being both deaf and bisexual—being forced to hide who and what he was, in a world that wanted anything that wasn't white, straight, rich, able-bodied, and preferably male to be squeezed out of the picture. Even Hollywood told Ray he'd never make it if he bared his hearing aid onscreen. Ray was never given the opportunity to present who he was to mainstream audiences, who he was when he performed on underground stages like the Flame Show Bar. In one interview from 1952, Ray referenced himself as a "freak." "They come to see what the freak is like! They want to know what this cat has got. I know what this cat has got. I make them feel. I disturb them. I exhaust them. I bring one or another of their buried controlled emotions to the surface." Even readers in the 1950s sensed that there was something about Ray, something that sat between the lines.

By 1953 Ray had turned his back on rock and roll just as Elvis, another white kid from the suburbs with Black sensibilities, appeared on the American music scene. People knew Ray had something to do with that; they all watched when America found their golden boy in the wailing riff of a white boy with a quiff. Poor Ray was left in the shadow of that spinning spark. Presley's sound was undeniably Black but it was more pronounced than Ray's in its masculinity. Elvis's influences were louder, less melancholic and more braggadocious. Elvis wore his influences, B. B. King and Rufus Thomas, on his dangled sleeve. A different tenor from Ray's influences, Billie Holiday and LaVern Baker. Ray's sound was gender-vague, a sound of ashtrays by the piano and lipstick on the mirror. He was an effeminate man and, for this time, challenged all the protected borders of identity. Ray may have been born too soon to receive mainstream appreciation but just the act of speaking about him now clarifies some glitchy ideas about our culture and the performative ways we treat race, disability, and sexuality.

Ray's management helped him set up a school for the deaf in 1953, when most deaf kids had nothing but bits of narrow roads in front of them. Ray would visit the school once a year after his tours and introduce himself to the students because he knew he could be a kind light for them. I imagine the deaf children were always in awe of him, but he didn't always stand so tall, sometimes he stumbled over his words and got embarrassed. His deafness was still a sensitive area of experience for him to manage and some of the kids bore it better and prouder than Ray. I imagine one of the deaf boys in the school, always asking other people to repeat or speaking some sign language that Ray never bothered to perfect, perhaps out of shame. Perhaps Ray didn't want to wear his deafness too loudly?

Shame. It's a thing that stings so many of us. At least Ray was trying, at least Ray showed up, at least Ray kept the lights on in the school by talking more publicly about his deafness. On *The Ed Sullivan Show* in 1956 he said that the school was close to his heart, but everyone knew Ray's heart was a dark and complicated place, a place where he struggled to speak.

Lotus wore tight fitted durags and a clunky backpack. He walked like a giant foot in the wrong shoe. He wore trousers tight on his waist and thick sweaters even in summer. He was hearing and I liked him. Lotus's voice was slightly nasal but it had depth.

And he was well spoken so he was easy to lip-read. This, combined with his mild manner, led to some of the other black boys calling him a "coconut"—the slang term for a person who is "black on the outside but white on the inside." I look less distinctively black—Lotus thought I was Italian when we first met—but I was nicknamed by some as "Dumb Boy," pronounced more like "dumbo," because of my hearing aids, or perhaps more creatively "Bush Boy" because I grew my hair out so it would cover my ears.

We were the kind of boys who wrestled for hours after watching *WrestleMania,* grappling each other with the moves of our favorite muscled men, sleeper holds and clotheslines, falling flat on our backs together. We were the kind of boys who saw any wide-open space and turned it into a ring.

One sunlit afternoon Lotus and I wrestled on the glowing grass by the basketball court between our blocks. The sun was high and the sound of the birds in the one tree made it feel like a forest. I took my hearing aids out and nestled them in our pile of shirts. We wore vests and our skin was smoother than a quiet river.

Holy . . .

Slim.

Dark.

Holy . . .

Two brown-black boys wrestling in the sun.

Holy . . .

He had me pinned to the ground, we grunted over each other, our bodies almost stuck together as we rumbled. Wanting the other to submit, to surrender, to hurt but not scar or draw blood. We didn't break eye contact, it assured us that we were safe in each other's grip, we were in control as we held each other on the warm grass through each improvised movement.

Holy . . .

An older boy, darker than Lotus and me, walked onto the basketball court in blue baggy shorts, saw us grappling on the ground. "Man, you have no idea how gay you look." Lotus stood up, straightened his vest. I stayed on the ground. "Man, fuck you," Lotus said, and the grass stopped glowing.

Lotus invited me to his house after school. We stayed in his room listening to music. He made hip-hop beats on his computer and was playing them to me. Mid–head nod I pointed at the handkerchiefs by his bed and laughed. "You don't have a cold, bitch," I said, then jumped on him and put him into a sleeper hold. His room was in his parents' attic, concealed white walls and wooden window frames, like a stylish tree house. It smelled of leaves and washing powder. It got late and he said I should stay over. I slept on a mattress on the floor next to his bed.

Hours after falling asleep in Lotus's room with my hearing aids under my pillow, I woke without opening my eyes, lying on my back. I felt a hand on my groin moving toward my shaft. The hand undid one of the buttons on my boxers. I lay still a moment, needing to be sure what was happening; I could hear blood pulsing in my head. I felt the hand try to pull my shaft out but I shot up in the bed and briefly saw the dark outline of Lotus, leaning over me. He flew backward like a shadow had slammed his body onto his mattress. He lay still, pretending he was asleep in his bed, quiet as land by a lake. I lay there listening to the blood in my head until my mouth was cold and dry from my heavy breath, then I hurried, dressed, grabbed my hearing aids from under my pillow, and, without putting them in and making no effort to be quiet, I rustled and thumped and scraped through the house and left.

On my way home from Lotus's house I kept checking my watch as I waited for the night bus: 4:12 A.M. It felt like a new time zone. My mind split from my body, I kept replaying over and over what happened. It rewound and played, rewound, played, and then became a *WrestleMania* action replay; actions I wished I'd taken grew in violence: a knee in his nose, a fist in his eye, a chair over his head. At school I told Emanuel, a mutual friend of ours, what he did, expecting wise words from him. He was the only boy who could grow a full beard. But his projected wisdom failed me; he was just a boy like any of us. He would stir and shit-talk for pure entertainment and each time he told someone about what had happened the rumor would slowly slant into new angles.

"I didn't do that, bro," said Lotus, who'd used all his breath that day defending himself to our other friends, and then to the strangers from other year groups who had started calling him "Lotus Pokus." Lotus yelled, pointing at me, "He's the gay boy! He touched me!"

"Swear down," said Ben, an older boy, outside the science block with a basketball under his arm. "If my mate touched me in my sleep he'd be fucking dead. You best put some serious bruises on him."

No one in our world believed back then that boys like me who are easily talked into violence are part of a patriarchal problem: an idea of power, an image of control and capability, something that proved I was a tough, real man. In truth, I was an insecure boy with something to prove, willing to do one mindless thing that could harden my entire life.

Here's the thing: I didn't know any other stories that could help or speak to what was happening in my life, but they must have been out there, there must have been stories about boys like us, deaf, queer, whatever, but where were they? How could I find them? How could I stitch them together and make a kind of sense, even when they contradicted each other; how could they sing, dance, square up?

In a 1977 TV interview, when the interviewer Hugh Downs refers to Ray's deafness as a "handicap," Ray chuckles and quickly corrects him. "You mean a hearing aid!?" Ray seems more relaxed with himself as an older man and is finally able to assert his relationship with his deafness.

"It's not a handicap," says Ray, slightly smirking. "When I go to bed and the phone rings, maids vacuum, there's knocks on doors . . . I don't hear any of that so I get lots of sleep that way."

One of my favorite performances by Johnnie Ray is his 1955 self-penned hit "Paths of Paradise." It's a skilled piece of songwriting too, full of careful and surprising phrasing despite all the end rhymes. For me, it has a hint of a bluesy "Sea of Love"–era Phil Phillips, a glam-rock Tom Waits, and a *Ladies' Man*–era Leonard Cohen in it.

In the video, Ray leans against a window in his lavish apartment, sobbing into his arm. We see Ray from the side; his hearing aid is bared to the camera as he gently pounds the window with his fist. He is wearing a suit and tie. A sad string section and horns lift and a ghostly harmony warbles in the background, just in time for Ray to turn around; scowling melodramatically at the camera, he sings . . .

"Last night I dreamed I walked along the paths of paradise . . ."

As Ray slinks around the apartment, we're given the scale of it: a large desk and record player by the door, a harp stands right by the window next to a painting of a violin, a white-cushioned chair in one corner, a grand piano in another.

You might be reminded of the scene in 1941's *Citizen Kane,* with Orson Welles as Charles Foster Kane, a wealthy businessman left lonely and heartbroken after his wife leaves him, standing alone in his extravagant echoing mansion, Xanadu.

Ray shows an incredible vocal range in this song; he belts high and low, whispers, whimpers, and screams. The performance is an aesthetic hybrid, part musical theater, part ballroom crooner, part cloak-and-dagger opera, part pretty-boy pop and smooth-faced, blue-eyed soul.

There's a freedom in this performance that is striking; despite how wildly he flails his arms, he never loses control of his voice, it's just his body that can't contain his large feelings.

As Ray builds toward the end of the song, his words tumble but they always land clear and perfectly on beat.

Just before he wails, his eyes glare up at the spotlight that shines brightly on his face; he quickly spins his body around before finishing the line and the note:

". . . to walk again the paaaaatttthhhh of parrrraaaadiiiissss-eeeee."

And here, we're left looking at Ray's back, but it's such a magnificent performance that I can only imagine him smiling to himself, privately grinning, taking out his handkerchief, wiping away the sweat running down the side of his face, whispering to himself,

Ray . . .

that was a good one.

9

Words, Signs, and the Critical Voice

Was it the early nineties when my parents took me on an anti-apartheid march on Parliament Square? Two poets sharing the stage, a tall dreadlocked man with a gap-toothed smile, Benjamin Zephaniah, and a tall gray-haired man with stern, thoughtful eyes, Adrian Mitchell. I didn't have hearing aids yet, I couldn't make out the words, but with both these poets on the stage, gazing over the gathered crowd, even the Houses of Parliament shrank behind them as Adrian chanted, "Tell me lies about Vietnam!" and Benjamin pleaded, "Open up yuh mind!" through a white-and-red megaphone.

Years later, was it John Agard in the black radical bookshop Centerprise in Dalston, leaning forward in his chair, porkpie hat, scruffy stubble beard, who blared, "Mi checkin' out mi history!"? Was it Jean "Binta" Breeze sitting outside the Hackney Empire smoking a roll-up, my mother pointing at her as we walked past, saying, "We have her book on our shelf!"?

What I can say for certain is that the poem "London" by William Blake was pasted on my bedroom wall, and I can cite the whole poem from memory, from the chartered streets to the marriage hearse. I can say for certain that "The Song of the Banana Man" by Jamaican poet Evan Jones, pasted on the wall on my mother's staircase, was the first poem I recited at school. From the "tourist white man wipin' his face" to the praising "of God and his big right hand I will live and die a banana man." I can say for certain that it was my mother who put "If We Must Die" by Jamaican poet Claude McKay under my eye when she saw that we were studying the Second World War in school, the hearsay that Winston Churchill's famous speech had lifted elements from this poem, the charged sonnet, the defiant "dying, but fighting back"; I can say for certain that this captured much of the sound in my imagination.

Around 2004, the year my friend Greg and I joined Kings Gym, a bodybuilding gym in Bethnal Green, our walls were full of posters of beefy masculine muscled celebrities. LL Cool J, Will Smith, Vin Diesel. I started buying protein supplements; within a year I'd gained forty-two pounds in muscle. Greg took me on his motorbike to and from the gym; I was spending more time at his house, playing N64 games and listening to music. I dropped my DJ Check and DJ Check Mate radio show, dropped swimming and the football team I played for on the weekend.

Everything was focused on bodybuilding and listening to hip-hop and rap, while privately I was filling up notebooks with dense and loose associative imagery that I wasn't calling poetry but "words."

I wrote a lot in my "words" notebooks and began posting some of it on an internet forum called "RapFlava." My mum bought a dial-up modem so I didn't have to leave the house for internet access. A few months before, at Hackney Community College, I had got up from my computer to use the photocopier and when I returned a boy had closed all the windows on my screen and opened the internet, playing a music video. I'd never seen him before. Immediately I saw he had two other boys beside him. Adrenaline tightened my whole body: a fast feeling of invincibility. I refused to back down.

I saw a flash of silver, something I thought was a metal ruler or a math compass, and he plunged it into my right leg. I didn't feel any pain at first. As security guards rushed into the room, I stood up straight, dizzy and high, shouted something like *fucking pricks,* and checked my ear. The single hearing aid I'd been wearing had fallen off somewhere. I looked on the ground, under the desk. Then I saw the damp patch of blood on my leg. Then the pain roared and I passed out.

I was lucky the blade missed the artery. I was barely conscious while police questioned me and asked me to make a statement so they could file a report. Hearing aid–less, I let the questions wash over me. It was clear the officers assumed I was part of the local gang. This allowed them to spare me their sympathy, their tone accusatory. Perhaps they were just jaded from the job, had already seen too much. When they asked if they could search my things, they found nothing in my bag but books and pens, nothing in my pockets but my own blood.

I never returned to the college and I didn't tell my mother about any of this. I told her I was staying with a friend while I was in the hospital, then, once I was healed enough to walk without limping I stayed at her house and buried myself in an online writing community.

Ayan 633
Sick bro!

Jive___02
Deeeeeeep!

I-Used-2-Luv-Her
Ah, I see hw u goin' on, nah can't lie, this is powerful.

These were my first readers, kind, supportive, anonymous strangers. I kept posting and giving equally positive critique to others who were sharing lyrics and poems.

My favorite member on RapFlava was called Avarice. He posted narrative poems about soldiers in war, friends in his neighborhood; some of the speakers in the poems were Mexican, Latino, and black. I sent poems I'd studied at school—"War Photographer" by Carol Ann Duffy and "Checking Out Me History" by John Agard—to Avarice's DMs to see what he thought. He sent back his favorite lines and seemed to appreciate the discussions.

Eventually I told my mum about Avarice's poems and showed

some of them to her, opening the window on the screen. She leaned over my shoulder, muttering the words out loud.

"He's good, isn't he?"

As a teenager I was still writing privately at night; during the day I was in the workforce losing numerous jobs on zero-hour contracts, meaning my employers had no obligation to offer me minimum hours. I worked in warehouses, removals, courier companies, hotels, etc. Each job ended in a similar way: someone in a suit shaking their head after telling me to do something, and finding I'd done the opposite because I hadn't heard all the instructions.

"We better get this guy something else to do," said yet another manager behind a desk, but they wouldn't get me something else to do. They just wouldn't call me back.

One of the last zero-hours jobs I got was working as a hotel receptionist. After a month I was called into the manager's office for a "disciplinary hearing." Ironic for a deaf person. I had no idea what I'd done wrong.

I sat in a small office on a hard wooden chair while my manager, a woman in her early forties with long blond hair and large blue eyes, clasped her hands on the desk in front of her.

"People have noticed how you sit behind reception idly while the phone rings and rings." I nodded, explained that I was "a bit deaf." She responded by saying that I didn't seem deaf and that I hadn't stated it on my CV or in my interview for the job.

"It's not a good sign," she said, her hands still clasped together, another ironic thing to say to a deaf person. "Customers think we don't care about them if they see us ignoring other customers." I nodded, said nothing; she continued. "I've even had a few complaints that some say hello and you don't return their greetings."

My manager had not noticed that I had been wearing one hearing aid—even though I needed two, but one made me look less deaf. She had never noticed it and now she looked concerned.

"Also, I've seen you writing in a notebook while on shift. I'm not convinced you want to be here."

I was given one more chance and told to wear both hearing aids.

That chance was blown the following week. A woman had come to the reception desk to complain about the temperature of the pool downstairs; apparently it was two degrees too cold. I had locked myself in a cubicle on a "toilet break" to write and had lost track of time.

When I returned to reception the manager was standing there with two women in their fifties with dyed black hair and heavy-set faces, in white lavender-scented robes, snarling at the manager: "Oh, here he is!"

The manager saw my notebook in my hands and the ink stain from a busted Biro on my suit trousers. She shook her head.

One of the women fixed her eyes on me with intense disdain that I had kept her waiting, that she'd had nowhere to direct her urgent complaint about the two-degree-too-cold pool water. "Look at you, no wonder you're just a receptionist." The manager called me into her office, asked me to leave. "You're the worst employee I've ever had."

Desperate to get away I searched for voluntary work and ended up overseas, in Ohio in the United States, volunteering as a camp counselor, working with young people and supervising sports activities. It was here that I worked with deaf young people and CODAs (children of deaf adults); it was here I met deaf people who laughed at me, seeing all the comedy in a deaf person pretending they could hear.

"Counselor Ray! I feel sorry for you!" signed a deaf ten-year-old boy, standing at the top of a waterslide while I was lifeguarding. "You're deaf and you can't sign! Ahahhahaha!" He did a kind of Charlie Chaplin impression, then shot down the slide, still laughing. "Ahahhahahahha!"

I couldn't follow his American Sign Language because it is almost completely different from British Sign Language.

ASL is rooted in French Sign Language, brought to the United States by Deaf French immigrants who settled in America. BSL is indigenous to the UK; the oldest illustrations of the BSL alphabet are over five hundred years old. The BSL alphabet is on two hands, ASL is on one.

Throughout my working trip I kept my "words" notebook; in it I wrote streams of conscious thoughts. One evening I left it out and one of the CODA kids saw it, read a bit of it, then handed it to me.

"Cool, you're a poet, you write poetry."

This was the first time someone called me a poet. It was like a spell, a summoning, and it refocused me, my life, my writing, my words becoming poetry.

On my last week of camp I was invited to a bar in downtown Columbus, Ohio, that hosted a talent contest. A man got up and read a poem into the microphone. I was startled, seeing the thing I had instinctively been doing since I was six, writing things down and reading them out. The public modeling of this fused connections I had yet to make between the space of private and public poetry.

One of my friends from Fortismere reached out to invite me to a poetry and music night at The Spitz in Shoreditch.

We stood at the front, glaring up at the stage at a blokey Cockney with short brown cropped hair, a long brown coat, and boots, part punk, part rockabilly. His name was Tim Wells. He read poems that referenced the Wailers, Joe Strummer, fighting Thatcher, but woven into these sounds and sentiments was a tender poem about his grandmother. His voice was strong in the mic but I still pushed my hearing aids into my ears and turned them up, not wanting to miss a word. Tim did look like the kind of man that hid a baseball bat up his trench coat, which made the tenderness of some of his poems even more moving to me.

The next poet was Chris Redmond, who performed a poem about the demolition of a tower block in Hackney, something I too remembered seeing; he'd woven it into a poem about seeing James Brown perform live.

The poet after that was a skinny pencil-shaped man with a huge black beard and a baseball cap. People were chatting, bar noises swirling. I turned my hearing aids down . . .

The pencil-shaped man pulled a stack of paper out of his suit jacket and exclaimed:

"THIS IS A LETTER . . ."

The bar fell immediately silent.

"FROM GOD TO MAN."

He read on, keeping the audience in complete stillness; you could feel the listening. His name was Scroobius Pip.

After the reading I spoke to Tim, Chris, and Scroobius Pip. They were friendly and I asked how I could find places where people wanted to hear poems. They all pointed me to the Poetry Café in Covent Garden.

I began attending open mics at the Poetry Café in winter 2007. It was a regular haunt of open-mic poets, the launch pad for many poets cutting their teeth on the London poetry circuit. Tuesday nights were Poetry Unplugged, the most popular of all the open mics, hosted by the poet Niall O'Sullivan in a downstairs basement bar. It became my gateway to the world of live poetry performance.

Sound-wise the basement was tricky to manage—it took a few weeks for me to work out the best place to situate myself so I could hear. It had a hardwood floor and low ceiling space; sound was solid and didn't bounce as long as I was at the front. The biggest hurdle was the steep rickety staircase on the side of the room. No one could get down it quietly; the sound of feet stamping down the stairs took over everything.

After that I heard about poetry slams from a promoter at the Poetry Café, a tall headmastery-looking man with bushy gray hair and a piece of spit that never left the side of his mouth.

My first slam, I waited agitated in my seat for my name to be called. "Please welcome Educated Fool!" I wore a hoodie and baggy jeans, kept a stiff serious face, and shouted my first line. A heartbreak poem I had written after my first girlfriend left.

"LAST NIGHT I MISSED YOU!"

The audience seemed to freeze, as if my voice was an alarm and they weren't told how to respond.

"LAST NIGHT I HUGGED MYSELF AND KISSED YOU!"

My mouth was too close to the mic and it kept popping on the s's, sounds I don't hear without amplification but in the mic became punctures in the air.

"LAST NIGHT WAS LONELY UNTIL I MINGLED . . ."

I only had one hearing aid in out of self-consciousness. I didn't want to be read as deaf.

". . . WITH ALL THE DREAMS THAT ARRESTED YOU, MY SOUL IS THE LOST TIME I INVESTED IN YOU!"

The intensity I brought to the stage had no air, no breathing; it was stifled angst finding its way out of my head.

"NEVER KNEW I'D BE LEFT, DESTITUTE

NEVER KNEW THAT TO THINK OF YOU IS ALL I'M LEFT TO DO

NEVER KNEW I'D DISCOVER THAT YOU WERE NEVER TRUE

BECAUSE YOU TURNED AND DID EVERYTHING

YOU SWORE YOU'D NEVER DO."

First time publicly speaking these words felt like finding a good place to scream, like much of my suppressed anxiety and angst could be released, acknowledged, and, if lucky, applauded.

My voice was something I was trying to hone, something that was seeking a certain approval. This was heightened by my years of speech therapy and my need for others to recognize my intelligence. Privately and now publicly, poetry held and honored many of my own burdens and truths; it felt like I was on my way to a lasting world of revelatory liberation and I refused to lose my path to it.

I got to the final and was beaten by a poet even younger than me, Deanna Rodger. A mixed-race seventeen-year-old who delivered her lines on tiptoes, reaching out to the air in front of her as if the words were precious jewels she was trying to bring back. She had a naturally well-pronounced voice, an instrument she played from the gut. Even the words I missed had a musicality that bore feeling.

Another time, I was sitting in the audience at the Poetry Café, when my hearing aid batteries died, both of them almost at the same time. The poet on the stage was a short, gaunt man with patchy gray hair and a baggy blue creased shirt. He used the word "talisman" (a word that eluded me at school too) as a refrain, but without amplification I heard the word as "tal-man" or "tally man"—the "is" sound needed to prop up the meaning and gesture of the poem was lost to me. Then, I heard the word "talisman" in a way that made no sense: "scalp"? "help"? Busy with the puzzle of sound and meaning, externally I smiled, applauded, and projected enjoyment and comprehension, perhaps nodding a bit too hard, "mm-ing" a bit too loudly. The poet got to the end of his poem and looked rattled by my audience noise, scowling in the spotlight. "This fake appreciation is annoying!" he ranted into the mic. "You don't have to pretend something is funny or that you're enjoying something, you don't have to make my poem about you, just be quiet and try to have a real response to the poems." Shamed by his critique, I bit my lip the rest of the night, sunk in my dulled sound, wondering if I was capable of a real response.

Navigating the sound in venues became a huge invisible part

of being a poet. I would show up early and walk around the spaces and suss out where best to stand. Often it was at the front to the side, next to the speaker farthest from the entrance. If that seat wasn't available I would slink to the next closest space and often I sat only half hearing the poems, smiling whenever laughter erupted at a joke everyone else seemed in on and I just wanted to blend into it.

The worst venues were the clubs and pubs that had their bar near the stage, the people behind the bar with cocktail shakers not even waiting for poems to finish, just shaking over the words. I would stare at them, my newest enemies, my constant nemeses. It was beyond my imagination for poetry nights to have captions or interpreters, I had to work with the ears I had.

By now I was performing anywhere that welcomed poets—comedy clubs, pubs, bars, teahouses, nightclubs, as well as slams in theaters and at universities.

Sarah, a consultant who worked for the nonprofit poetry organization Apples and Snakes, had seen me at a poetry night in Tottenham alongside a rising star on the scene, Michaela Coel. I hadn't realized it was a Christian poetry night until the poets in the lineup included Bible passages and reminders that "Jesus sees all," which would inspire the loudest cheers. My poetry set bombed. I wasn't advocating for the Lord and Savior Jesus Christ, I was performing shouty secular poems that quoted Malcolm X, Bob Marley, and William Blake, poems that preached "the light located within."

Sarah offered me a mentor to develop my writing. The first

poets I asked to be mentored by were Benjamin Zephaniah and Lemn Sissay, and I would have asked for Adrian Mitchell but he had died. None were available. She paired me with Guyanese Grenadian British poet Malika Booker, who ran a community space for poets called Malika's Poetry Kitchen and was known to nurture mainly working-class and black poets.

Over the next six months I met with Malika at the National Poetry Library in London's Southbank Centre. Green-carpeted with dim flashing strobe lighting, shelves in aisles that had to be cranked open, the glass door entrance opened silently, everything opened silently. I turned off my hearing aids as soon as I entered. The spectacled librarians in cotton sweaters and cardigans shuffled with books toward the stacked shelves, rule keepers, no laptops on the desks; they'd appear quietly over your shoulder to check that you were writing poetry and not doing university coursework or accounts, nothing but poetry permitted. My liberation was gently and sternly authorized by these wizardly poetry librarians.

Malika's first question to me was: "What are you reading?" I heaved my bag onto the table like it was full of rubble and placed each book on the table, among them *The Autobiography of Malcolm X* and Che Guevara's *Motorcycle Diaries*. I read books that quoted poetry but not actual poetry books. I was stumped; I'd never thought of poetry collections, just individual poems. Malika gave me time to explore the library shelves, to flick through pages of poems and find verses to read to her.

I picked up a book by Canadian poet Mark Strand and read a poem called "Mirror," about a man at a party who notices a mirror in which he sees a woman at the far end of the room. The poet speculates on the woman's story and its possible symbolism while wondering what exact "shade of yellow the setting sun turned our drinks." We spoke about that poem as a "narrative" poem, the distillation of language to its pure form, which is what the light is also doing to the drink in the poem. Malika taught me about images in poems, how one image follows another, about what Derek Walcott said about the link between prayer and poem, to avoid mixing metaphors and, most importantly, to read widely. Read poets in translation as well as those writing in English.

In Russian poet Vladimir Mayakovsky's work, I discovered a poet with volume on the page. You could hear the intensity of his voice as you read it. In his portrait on the cover of *Night Wraps the Sky,* Mayakovsky's eyes growl as a rolled-up cigarette dies between his lips, one side of his shaved head appears in shadow, his ear naked, openly facing us as fiercely as his tight scowling jaw.

"A Cloud in Trousers" (1914) is a thirty-page poem written in short, energetic lines of lyrical dialogue and proclamations, part soliloquy, part lyric love poem. The images often descriptions of gestures that sometimes read as stage directions.

Attention!
Ladies and Gents!

. . .

Have you seen
What's most frightening of all—
My face when I am
Absolute calm

The poem was so powerful I had to speak it aloud. I sat in the farthest corner of the library with my hearing aids off, reading out the lines. I saw how Mayakovsky's words filled stadiums, how he encapsulated a loudness, a literary style that was masculine and embodied "100 percent man"; he declares to a potential lover,

Maria
I ask for your body.

Years later, the first time my poetry was broadcast on BBC Radio 4, I stood onstage in front of a live audience in the Water Rats venue in King's Cross. I recorded a new poem, the only poem I had written about deafness, called "A Hard Act to Follow."

I began the poem intentionally mumbling, speaking quiet gibberish, progressively getting louder, no words decipherable. I paused, then announced the opening line:

Sometimes conversation is a hard act to follow.
Sometimes he doesn't quite catch what is said
But whatever it was he nods his head, says
Yesss?

The poem, like Mayakovsky's, is full of gestures and descriptions that could be read as stage directions.

Sometimes he says things that have already been said.
Sometimes he says things that have already been said.

And no one assumes he didn't hear them, instead
It's assumed he's stupid, clueless.

After two takes of the poem, the producer called me backstage after the recording.

"We have a problem," he said. "Your voice, these words"—he pointed at a list of words he'd written on his paper (I can't remember what they were). "You slur them, don't fill them out correctly. I can't use this poem."

The producer knew I wore hearing aids but he hadn't taken into account how that might make me sound and how it affects speech. The producer's words were traumatizing, pulling me back to school. Had I got it wrong, had Renata in fact failed me? Left me with unrefined, slurry speech?

I turned to Gee, the presenter, panicking, thinking I was about to lose my chance to be broadcast.

"Give me your notebook, everything you've written," said Gee and marched off with it. Half an hour later he returned holding my notebook open, pointing at a short, hurriedly composed poem I'd written about a tree. "We're going to record that." It had been decided the words in that poem were pronounceable. I did it in one take.

Afterward, distraught, I stopped showing up to gigs, paranoid my "slurry words" were exposing me. How could I be on a radio show if I sounded deaf? If I couldn't speak properly? If hearing people would judge my speech?

I sought out a speech therapist a week later at the Royal National Throat, Nose and Ear Hospital, coincidentally a few doors down from the Water Rats venue. She was a short brunette woman with a pointed nose. She had me read and repeat words, showing me some of the gaps in words I was missing, filling them in. We paused on the word "criticism." It was impossible for me to say wholly, it had disappearing sounds in it, sounds I couldn't hear. The "is" vanished next to the harder "ic" sound. I heard it as "cr-it-im." I practiced the sound of the word on my tongue and teeth, familiarizing myself with the shape and feel of the sounds to ensure I was shaping them out. She gave me a list of other words to practice. Our sessions were once a month, and by the end I was able to relay more tongue twisters, reframing the producer's criticism.

Recently, my son sat in his high chair at the breakfast table, staring out the window, intensely sucking his thumb, his whole face rattled with worry. "Are you okay, baby?" I asked. He popped his thumb from his mouth. "Dream. Scary!" he proclaimed, eyebrows raised, eyes unblinking. "You had a scary dream?" I asked, focusing on his language instead of his experience, rephrasing his words instead of asking him what the scary dream was. He repeated, this time with annoyance, "Dream! Scary!" I then used a word that he had not. "You had a nightmare, baby?" Now he looked lost, even more frustrated. As he sucked his thumb he began pinching his neck, something he does for comfort, but it wasn't working. He shrieked in one breath, "DREAM SCARY!" This time I leaned toward his body, calmly repeating his words, "Dream. Scary," and I used a word and a sign that I knew he knew: "sad." My son turned his gaze from the window and met my eyes, calmed, repeated the words and the sign, "Dream. Scary. Sad."

He was not asking for correction or constructive criticism. He was, instead, asking me to acknowledge his experience; he needed reassurance, that he is not wrong to feel what he feels, nor is he wrong to say it how he says it. It made me think of my younger (deaf) speech and how that producer's problem was not that my speech wasn't understandable, it was that it didn't sound proper, familiar, rounded out like a hearing person, or the poet-voice of a hearing poet.

Poet Holly Pester writes in her essay "The Politics of Delivery (Against Poet-Voice)" that "delivery [vocalizing a poem] is an opportunity to continually reassess the integration of one's self with speech." She goes on to ask, "Can intonated delivery be heard as a comment and critique of institutions that produce and oppress speaking subjects?"

Perhaps, if my deaf speech (or "poet-voice") was framed from day one as an accepted aesthetic, understood and broadcastable, perhaps I would have been a deaf poet living on lighter air, broken free from the kind of voice that willfully partakes in a codified system of structural inequality.

Dream? Scary? Sad?

10

Coming In from the Cold

How do you dress for your father's funeral? I'm wearing his bright orange blazer, thick padded shoulders, moth-eaten on the inside. I'm sitting in the backseat of the black Volvo next to my mother and sister, Marley wails through the iPad on my lap. The sky is white and sealed over by cloud. I ask the driver to stop outside the William Hill bookmakers where Dad gambled on the horses. I spent years walking to William Hill, the only other place I would find my father if he wasn't in his council flat.

I walk into the betting shop and my dad's friends are there. Ninja is the name of one of them, for reasons unknown to me, that is what everyone calls him. He is a short, bald black man with a slightly squashed face and thick patches of gray beard that move around his mouth when he talks. Most of what he says is incoherent mumbling because half of his teeth are missing. Then there's Desmond, a slightly taller, lighter-skinned man in a cream-colored jacket and light brown bowler hat; and Barry, a tall, slender black man in a white Puma T-shirt, a smart black blazer, a red baseball cap, and a gray goatee.

All are standing in front of the TVs. These were the West Indian men Dad would sit around the table with, drinking, laughing, and shouting at the horses. If they'd forgotten about the funeral, my bright orange blazer with my dad's folded handkerchief in my breast pocket reminds them. "Yuh old man funeral today!?" says Ninja, then calls the other men over. "Dis Seymour's son." The men gather around and shake my hand. "Him gone, him gone, but him still here." I look up at the TVs as the gates open and the greyhounds shoot from their cages. I walk to the counter and put down a fiver on a dog. I doubt whether Dad would be surprised that his friends at the bookmakers would miss his funeral. I take the betting slip and leave my dad's friends shouting at the row of screens.

At Manor Park Cemetery some friends and cousins I haven't seen in years show up. Everything about them belongs in the past. There is a Jamaican flag over my father's casket. My sister and I give speeches.

She'd stopped talking to Dad the night he showed up at the house drunk, and my sister had to defend our mother. She picked up two bricks from the garden and swung them in his face and fractured his jaw. My dad couldn't speak for a month without the pain connecting him to that night. My sister was fifteen and was forced to grow up quickly so she could help raise me and support our mother. She might always be resentful of that, but her speech is gentle and diligent; she trembles through it. My pain is watching her, the strongest woman I know, become a hurt child once again, keeping her head up for her brother, her mother, herself. I look out over the crowd at my scattered Jamaican relatives, different families sitting in their own sections of the church. My dad lost contact with many of the families years ago and that distance expresses itself in their positions, how far back they are sitting.

I tell the congregation: "I have yet to find a Jamaican restaurant that can make ackee and saltfish, breadfruit, green banana with rice and peas like my father. He would always give me a spoon to eat with and call me 'white bwoy' if I asked for a fork."

Everyone in the church laughs except the priest, who is the whitest man in the world.

"My father lived to seventy-five. He was a smoker, a drinker, and a gambler; my theory of his longevity is his sense of humor. Every joke he made gave him back the three minutes of life he lost to a cigarette. Not all his jokes were even funny: I remember sitting on the train with him at Dalston Kingsland; he said, 'Did I ever tell you the funny story about the suicidal train driver who drove his train into a station and killed a hundred people? Hee-hee-haha.' I said, 'Dad, that's not funny, why are you laughing?' and he'd say, 'What you want me to do, cry?' and he'd laugh again." The congregation laughs too. There's nothing like laughter at a funeral.

After the service everyone walks to the gravesite with the pallbearers, my cousins still keeping their distance. My dad's casket is lowered. I take out the betting slip and drop it into the earth.

I entered a state of numbness, in which sometimes sadness broke through and had me sobbing, convulsing. Everything around me was too familiar, everything meant too much, I knew that building, that street, that bench, that shopkeeper, everything that existed in a world my dad was once in and that was still standing when he wasn't. I booked a flight somewhere I had never been. Barcelona. It's warm, not too far away, and seemed to me a place to lose myself, to slow down and process grief. I rented an Airbnb, a one-bed tiny apartment on the top floor of a corner building. It looked out over the city of rooftops and narrow stone streets full of washing lines and dog walkers and cigarette smokers and lampposts; the Catalonian language that I couldn't enter chatted and babbled away in the bars and corridors as I walked through the city peacefully with my hearing aids off until I joined the queue outside the Basílica de la Sagrada Família, also known as Gaudí's cathedral. A tall, Gothic anciently futuristic temple that heaved into the sky like a huge concrete speech bubble from a long-dead God. I entered the tall heavy doors, paid for the audio guide, curious. I had my own powerful over-the-ears headphones, I inserted them into the audio guide tablet. I stood under a small unorthodox-shaped roof and pressed the audio guide on and turned the volume to maximum. The voice was male, clear with depth. It instructed me to look up and stare into the small enclosed section of the roof and shout and sing and be aware of how the sound of my voice moved into that space, how it expanded as it bounced off the walls. It reminded me of my speech therapist placing a bowl over my head and speaking to me, which meant hearing her more sharply because of how the shape of the bowl aided the route of sound into the brain. But this wasn't framed with the language of science, but spirituality. The audio guide described the experience of sound under that particular roof as divine, said that that was how angels experience sound, a vast vibrating white light of echoes. I knew there were sounds I couldn't pick up, dimensions that I couldn't enter. I wondered if we, deaf people, were included in this holy idea of sound, this portal, accessible from the ears. Over the next days, every street I walked down, every body of water I faced, every garden path I wandered through, that question kept ringing.

Eventually, when I had carried the question far enough, the air thinned, lightness arrived, sound settled, and I wrote ferociously into my notebook on the tables outside coffee shops and on a park bench beneath trees and in a bar on the stall by the window that shielded me from the busy outside world of traffic horns and voices and bicycle bells. I have never been able to write in silence, or when I'm feeling lonely. I need ambience, a feeling of life swathing around me, life that I can connect to as I find the language for it. Nothing makes me feel more capable.

By the time I left Barcelona I had the opening poem written of *The Perseverance,* titled "Echo," a channel for my grief, a way to tune in and sound it out. The feeling of numbness became a feeling of loneliness, a feeling of loneliness became a feeling of company; this is what the words were giving me.

Once, when I was months away from starting school, my dad won big on the horses. Betting on a twenty-to-one horse, he pocketed a wad of cash in an envelope, stuffed it into his inside coat pocket, and whistled out the bookie's door. He stopped by my mother's house, where he still had a key though they now lived separately, and walked into my bedroom.

"I'm taking us all to Jamaica."

His proud wide smile invited me into his arms.

Within months my parents, my sister, and I boarded an Air Jamaica plane from Gatwick for a two-week stay on the island. I was eleven or twelve. In Patty Hill, I met my grandmother Darcas, wheelchair-bound, for the first time. She had no teeth, skeletal; she sat facing the hills on her veranda, acknowledged me with a head nod while her jaw twitched as if she were constantly running her tongue along toothless gums. I wasn't wearing my hearing aids; I had kept them out after one of my cousins gawked without greeting me when I arrived. I didn't want to have to explain them and it seemed like there was a barrier between us so I kept them off. Sound was damper, thinner, but many Jamaicans project their voices, not shy with their interactions, which often felt stark and overbearing, harshly honest in ways that could be taken as cruel. I tried to lean away from the stings of judgments and surface impressions.

"Hin'nglish white bwoy, listen nuh? Yuh deaf bwoy, ta'rasss!"

Without my hearing aids I remained passive, letting anything wash over me, framing these interactions in my mind as surface, polite conversation, smiling, nodding.

My grandmother Darcas leaning her body toward me, saying: *WATA*.

I thought she was saying "What a . . ." and then not finishing her sentence . . .

What a what?

WATA!

Her eyes fixed on an empty glass on the table by her bed. I picked it up and went into the next room where there was a bucket of water. I scooped the cup in the bucket, knowing the water was freshly gathered from the waterfall up the hill, and came back, watched my grandmother gulp gulp down in one. She turned and she gave me the only smile she would give me in this life.

I met Aunt Avis, the woman who raised my father, in Kingston. I sat on her balcony, the same one where my father sat wailing through the white balcony bars for his father from half a century ago. Aunt Avis was full of life, talk talk, chat chat. I liked her but I also felt the weight of my father's silence around her. Aunt Avis talked a lot and my father seemed passive in comparison, nodding, smiling, evading anything that might overexpose him. He kept his hands busy, excusing himself from rooms to stand outside alone, smoking his roll-ups. I related to his silence.

On the plane to Jamaica for the first time since my father died, I was sitting next to a young white woman in short denim shorts; she put her bare feet up on the seat to varnish her toenails as the plane descended. I judged her brazenness. As she put her makeup away she pulled out her green Jamaican passport and placed it on the tray in front of her.

"You're a citizen?" I asked.

"Yes, I'm Jamaican, you?"

"My father was."

We exchanged stories, spoke about Jamaican progressiveness,

the ice cream at Devon House, the reliable service of the Knutsford Express (a bus that traveled all over the island), the expanding tech industry (Digicel, the company that had given the island stable Wi-Fi, etc.).

"So what's the benefit of having a British and a Jamaican passport?"

"When we leave the plane I'm going to get through a lot quicker than you."

"That's it?"

She shrugged.

After we touched tarmac at Norman Manley International Airport I was standing among the passengers at the baggage carousel. English tourists in floral shirts and sunglasses had already rubbed in their sun cream, ready to get to the hotel pools and private beaches, while everyone else heaved their overloaded luggage onto their backs, shoulders, and trolleys. It was clear who was on vacation and who was heading home.

Outside I was greeted by the driver, a man in a blue button-up shirt and a gold bracelet on his wrist.

As we drove into the center of town I saw a tall, white-haired man in a white linen outfit open the passenger door of his convertible, a fast-melting ice cream in his other hand. The woman in the denim shorts from the plane climbed into the car, her ice cream collapsing onto her painted fingernails.

The truth is I've never been able to relax in Jamaica; there's too much status anxiety infused with colorism and colonial baggage. The taxi drivers that seem keen to prove their Englishness to me with their football knowledge and some relative of theirs that lives on "Hox-ford Street," which often leads to a rant about Jamaican society being "better off under British rule," while I am quick to question the glorification of the English, keen to prove my Jamaican-ness and the "fuckery of Empire," but really we're both glaring through the tint at assumed greener grasses.

As a child I asked my dad why we didn't live in Jamaica. We were in Montego Bay, visiting Aunt Avis. I had spent days lying on the beach, snorkeling between coral reefs and translucent yellow fishes. We were on Aunt Avis's balcony looking over the mountains and all the shadows they cast.

"Limited," said my father, the same word he used to describe my deafness.

On my second day in Kingston I was interviewed on *Smile Jamaica,* a historic live morning TV show that lit up the small rectangular screen in my grandparents' living room in Patty Hill.

I was introduced to Antoinette Aiken, Jamaica's most prominent sign language interpreter. She stood interpreting in Jamaican sign beside the couch; the host had introduced me as a "so-called British Jamaican," then asked his first question:

"Are you Jamaican?"

Yes, my father was born here and I've been coming here since childhood.

The host sneered, leaning back, eyebrows raised.

"You're not Jamaican."

I felt the instant sting of the host vibrate in my chest. He went on:

". . . So they tell me that you're deaf but how are you deaf exactly? You don't look deaf, you hear me speaking now?"

This was essentially what that BBC host had said to me on

the radio months earlier. This is why I couldn't relax in Jamaica. This is why I couldn't relax in England. It's too easy to be spun away from any of the grounds I claim. Everything feels like it has to be earned, fought for, sussed out. I hadn't yet worked out how to not hear my father in every Jamaican man with a tendency to scorn and shame. The fact that the interview was broadcast live to the whole island meant going back to the hotel and not leaving again for the day.

What I came to remember is that Jamaica has a different rhythm and pace, it isn't personal. Conversation is often double-edged. To function I need to tune in to it. Western rhythm can't flow, it will keep me socially awkward and oversensitive; people's blunt comments need to wash over me, I need to pick them out of my skin and point them back.

This particular aspect of Jamaica makes deafness hard to assert; people often expect quick responses, there's little mercy given to accommodate anyone who moves slower, my listening strategy often doesn't work, people refuse to be inconvenienced by repeating themselves, and my light skin and British accent make some people automatically defensive, ready to fire. I cannot be read without the colonial gaze.

Once, as a child walking on a beach (without hearing aids in), a man with dreads and a string vest ran up to me, vexed.

"What the rassclaut you ignore me for, pussy boy!? You hear me, nuh? Mi call yuh from over dere."

I explained I was deaf; it seemed to make him angrier.

"Yuh pussy boy!" and he walked away, leaving me wondering what he wanted in the first place . . .

Then, a white man with a round stomach and a straw sun hat shouted from his hotel balcony:

What on earth are you doing talking to people like that, you moron?

The dread man looked up.

No sah, no sah, dat just how we talk talk inna island, Jamaican speak, mon.

I walked on as dread man apologized again to the sun hat man on the balcony.

The next morning I was driven to a local mainstream primary school in Kingston with a Jamaican-born novelist who now lives in New York and a young literacy advocate, also living in New York.

We stood in the assembly courtyard and took questions from students on poetry and living as a writer. One question asked of me by an eleven-year-old boy was:

"Is it emotional to write a book?"

I was moved by many of the thoughtful questions but that one stayed with me. I wasn't surprised, though: Jamaican students are typically high achievers. My cousin Shaun, who was born in New York and was a well-marked student in the United States, came to Jamaica and was so far behind in comparison to his peers that he had to repeat a year of school. All the students looked like they could be my cousins and nephews and nieces, so I felt a kind of pride and protectiveness.

I was asked to read a poem I'd written, a broken ghazal, "Jamaican British"—in the preamble I asked the class earnestly, "Where do you think I'm from?"

A resounding chorus of "WHITE!" erupted.

The other writers turned their heads, bursting out in laughter.

After the poem one of the teachers admitted to her students:

"I'm a light-skin Jamaican, born on the island, and I have to explain myself this way too."

After the assembly she shook my hand. "You remind me of my father. He was white," she said, tearing up.

At the Caribbean Christian Centre for the Deaf, I met Deaf Jamaicans who have developed a community that is also linked to Deaf Can Coffee, a nonprofit organization set up by Alfred Evelyn Clarke, a Deaf Jamaican farmer, which has helped teach young Deaf Jamaicans how to roast coffee beans. A number of Deaf Can coffee shops have now been launched around the island. Some deaf students at the school work in the coffee shops as baristas or teach some Jamaican Sign Language.

Antoinette Aiken, a CODA, gave me an anecdotal statistic: that 95 percent of people born deaf in Jamaica grow up illiterate. In the UK it's around 70 percent. Of course, this doesn't mean they grow up without language; rather, most would be functionally illiterate, meaning they could be fluent in sign language but struggle to write "grammatically correct" English.

The school was made up of cement buildings with zinc roofs surrounding a wide-open cement playground, where students were signing. The school's director was a Deaf Jamaican called Tashi Widmer; I walked into her office, shook her hand, and she signed her name. I had to quickly excuse myself from the room; something had erupted that I couldn't take. I trembled, trying not to burst, but it came, I couldn't stop it. I hadn't imagined this in Jamaica; I kept hearing my dead father's voice—"limited"—and I hadn't taken in my own limited imagination for what I could have become had I grown up in Jamaica, that existing on the island as a deaf person and thriving was possible, that connecting with my Jamaican family, blood and chosen, was possible, that having an integrated deaf identity on the island was possible.

The heat of that shame flooded me, the director held me, I cried, and she held me through the heat and convulsions while I apologized. "I'm sorry, I'm sorry, I'm sorry, I'm sorry, I just didn't know . . . I didn't know."

What I didn't know was that there was a place for me in Jamaica, that there were softer edges, a Jamaican deaf space where you weren't judged for having different needs, or assumed to be slow or uppity or whatever sharp projection came your way. I'd spent years unable to imagine what my acceptance in Jamaica could look like and, in a way, I'd found it, at least a part of it.

I gathered myself and ran a workshop in the school hall, asking if any of the class could show me a poem in Jamaican Sign Language.

A boy signed a Deaf fable of a lumberjack who tried to cut down a tree. When he shouted *TIMBER!* it wouldn't fall. A tree doctor tested the tree's hearing, said:

"This tree is deaf."

And he signed the word *TIMBER*

and the tree fell.

11

"What's Good About Being Deaf?"

I met Thomas when I was visiting a school in Durham in 2017. His teachers whisked me away after I delivered an assembly on poetry to a packed hall of eleven-to-sixteen-year-olds, to sit me in a room with him, a hazel-haired, round-headed eleven-year-old who had two large silver hearing aids in his ears. He kept his head down on the table as his teachers helicoptered over him. Thomas was the only deaf student in the school and the overzealous hearing teachers gathered Thomas and me in a quiet room to meet each other.

"So, Thomas," said one of the teachers, kneeling beside him. "This is a poet, he wears hearing aids like you." Another teacher butted in. "Yes, what do you have to say about being deaf, Thomas?"

None of the teachers knew sign; even the fact that sometimes they spoke without facing him showed me that Thomas wasn't in a room that was accommodating his needs. Thomas kept his head down and finally said, "It's useless."

I told Thomas that I felt useless at his age too, that I had internalized this idea that my deafness decreased my value and limited my future (employment and romantic). I explained that I had spent decades pushing against this notion. Deafness is harder when you have to rely on people who aren't deaf to understand you, people who don't have the patience to face you when they talk or speak sign, or know when to pause in conversation when there's a loud noise like an alarm going off or a truck bustling down the street. One of the teachers, perhaps feeling accused and that my words were negative, interrupted again. "Yes, but look at him, Thomas, he's now a famous poet." Thomas lifted his head from the table, stared at me, thinking, then asked, "Are poets useful?"

"Well," I said, "that's a good question, and intelligent people ask good questions." Thomas fidgeted with his thumbs. "I think there is a power in finding ways to articulate your unique self in the world, a useful power."

Poetry helped me, even if it was just a way to temporarily lift or lighten the narrative of the world, even if it didn't always transform my truths and traumas. At times it stopped me spiraling into the story of being that boy who stood low in rank along a long line of other boys who I thought were more clever, more beautiful, more rich, more worthy. I was the boy who wanted to blend in; blending in looked easier, calmer. I was the boy who didn't want to look like the enemy of any system, even a system that hated me, and I know I succeeded despite the system.

I thought of Thomas when I began doing readings of my first

children's picture book, *Can Bears Ski?,* a story based on my own experience growing up deaf with hearing parents who struggled to guide me through the hearing world. Part of the purpose of the story is to show deafness as an experience rather than a trauma. During those first readings I got a range of questions from deaf young readers. Some engaged with the story, asking, "Why does the moon have a face?" and, "Can the bears sign?" And there were young readers looking at the other faces on the Zoom call and asking, "How many people here have cochlear implants?" Another question was, "Does anyone here have red hearing aids?" but a common question I received was, "What's good about being deaf?" There is an innocence to this question, but there's also a self-consciousness, one that some would say ought to not exist for children so young, but, alas, from birth we're lucky to be born in a room that isn't ableist, let alone a world.

Forgive me, I'm not trying to be grandiose; I didn't mean for poetry to give me a platform for sweeping statements of self-affirmation. For a long time, my poetry was private, it helped me hide. I hid behind poetic thought, in part because it was an intellectual activity that asserted my potential usefulness. In reality, I had no idea what a deaf racially ambiguous boy could offer the "real" world.

The poet Deanna Rodger invited me to an event that combined human rights and immigration lawyers with writers and poets responding to the Brexit referendum results. The whole country seemed stunned. At least that was the temperature in London.

"What the fuck has he done, what the fuck has he done?" said a voice somewhere, perhaps in my head or from the open windows of the Hackney houses I walked by on my way to a gig at the Stuart Hall Library in Shoreditch. I sat at the front, nearest one of the speakers, as Deanna performed her "London" poem. I performed my "Jamaican British" poem and afterward, as the crowd trickled out of their seats, Deanna and I stood by the exit, greeting and giving farewells to people as they left, not unlike how my grandparents ended their church services, standing by the door, thanking the congregation for attending. A tall, light-skinned black woman with light brown curly hair and wide intelligent eyes approached Deanna. "I enjoyed your poem, thank you." She spoke in a somewhere-in-America accent, a clear voice full of gliding vowels; her sounds asserted themselves, projected confidence even as she shuffled away. Noting her American accent, Deanna reached out her arm. "Speak to Raymond, the other poet!" I had recently been in Chicago and was still jet-lagged. Her name was Tabitha. Deanna's introduction had us exchanging numbers, then dating, then kissing for the first time a week later, outside a bar in Holborn, rain pelting down. I leaned into her lips under an umbrella and months of love and companionship between us followed, made easier by the fact she was having to return to the States, meaning we could be casual and unrestrained. There was something about that dynamic that was liberating.

On early dates I noted that anything I didn't hear Tabitha say, she repeated without annoyance or exasperation. At a bar or restaurant, she never called across the table or the room, she came to me; she never called up the stairs or through the walls from another room, she came in before speaking. Her deaf awareness was coincidental; it aligned with her style of communication, her love language. She was present, engaged, a good listener.

On an early date, we were in Rudie's restaurant in Brixton, Tabitha was watching me eat, rushing my food as if in some private and restless race. She reached across the table, touched my hand, asked, "Are you here?" She asked it slowly, so slow it stopped my mouth and I began to taste the scrambled softness of ackee, the peppered brown rice and peas in the candlelight between us.

Tabitha invited me to New Orleans, her hometown, where her large family resides.

The city was almost unwalkable because of the highways and huge willow trees that bulge, pump, and pull up the ground, turning over the paving slabs by the roads that are already punctuated with potholes. It is as if the swampy natural world is pushing back against the concrete one. It's a city of multiplicity, nothing is one thing. Some of the porches outside the houses waved large New Orleans flags, two red and blue stripes between a larger white stripe with three yellow fleur-de-lis symbols in the middle—it's a remix of the French flag. The city is divided into parishes, just like islands in the Caribbean; large bursts of crows often appear in the skies, the Gothic cemeteries full of decaying stone angels that bow over the earth, facing the crumbling walls and the brown and white rusted gates, all of it once underwater, many of the buried bodies washed away somewhere. The twilight zone frequency of the city is easy to romanticize. It's a city in constant conversation with the dead and undead, never fully recovered from Hurricane Katrina. Tabitha lost family to that terror and was herself displaced. She told me that story and I found my listening change in New Orleans. It's a city deeply connected to its water; you have to know the nearest bridge over the river to locate yourself and others.

One night Tabitha took me to Bacchanal, a bar on the bywater near the railway tracks: All the drinks on the tables trembled as the freight trains rumbled past; a wavy-haired man in a purple shirt played the piano in front of us, beside him a bald-headed black man blowing a gold and shiny saxophone, a well-built black man in a black T-shirt on the drums, a white man in glasses and a blue blazer blowing a trumpet, and an afroed brown-skinned man on an upright base—they looked like college students but played like elder jazz musicians. They tapped, plucked, bounced, and weaved through each groove and I forgot where I was until the softer brushes, the spacey trickles, the quick high hats brought me back to the rhythm of the powerful river. Here, a piano key illustrated my deafness perfectly. All the music disappeared and the pianist had hit a single note. I heard the chord ding, then vibrate for a split second and stop, but it hushed the audience; everyone around me stopped and focused on the band, the vibration of that one note had disappeared, but looking around I could see everyone transfixed, activated in listening. I nudged Tabitha. "You hear that?" She nodded. "What do you hear?" I asked. "The piano key, it's still traveling." After a few more seconds I asked, "You still hear it?" "Faintly." My ears heard the full initial sound of the piano key but almost none of its aftermath, its reverberating resonance. I explained that experience to Tabitha's cousin Curtis; he smiled, said, "Well, it sounded like the sun setting over the Mississippi River, you should go see it tomorrow"—and the next day I stood on the bank at Algiers Point at 5:45 P.M. and looked toward the bridge, watching the sunset behind it, a sky of bright smoky coal-fire orange and red and pink and blue. I stared, missing none of it.

Later that night, Tabitha told me she loved me for the first time as we lay on the sofa in the living room of the rented purple house that looked out at the river. I didn't say it back. Not yet. I expected love to feel static, a place you couldn't move away from, something not second-guessable. But New Orleans was reminding me that there are many ways of holding things, with our ears, eyes, nose, tongue, skin, as well as the things that seem beyond us, like intuition. I was too high to land on any words anyway, too warm with new feelings to name what was stirring me. Everything I was sensing while living beside the Mississippi River was about movement, never arrival.

Two years later, Tabitha and I married by the Mississippi River. After the reception it begins to rain hard. Tabitha said she had an urge to drive to the neighborhood her grandmother, dead seven years, had lived in; she swore the rain had a message in it, swore she heard her grandmother calling, swore she needed to take me to the river to meet her. Tabitha drove downtown and parked and we walked, rain still pelting down. She faced the dark water and I could feel the presence of Tabitha's grandmother in the rain. I couldn't see her, but I could; I couldn't hear her, but I could.

Palestinian teacher of the deaf Hashem Ghazal—a leading figure at Atfaluna Society for Deaf Children, an ambassador for Deaf culture and disability justice, often called Gaza's "Godfather of the Deaf," and father to nine children (six of them born deaf)—

delivered a TedTalk in 2015 entitled "Let the Fingers Do the Talk," in the Shujaiya neighborhood in Gaza City.

Throughout the presentation, Ghazal details anecdotes from his life, from his father's passing at a young age, the challenges he faced in his childhood as a deaf youngster, and learning carpentry. He explains how he had to advise his deaf children, to let them know what is good about being deaf; he had to sign to them, saying not to be ashamed of deafness, that "this is a destiny from God, and God has compensated us with the language of speech and sign." There is a deep need for deaf communities everywhere to have empowering figures like Ghazal, people who understand, through their own experience, how harsh the world can be to the deaf.

In 2024 Ghazal was murdered in an IDF airstrike on Gaza alongside his wife. I had hoped to meet him and make a documentary on his work for the D/deaf, a figure who lived the question and the answer, the good of being D/deaf; someone I could point to for Thomas, for us all.

12

Sounding Out

A study recently conducted at King's College London suggested that people who live in close proximity to birds, birdsong, trees, and sky within a city are thought to be happier than those who don't. I think about this often, because my ears miss the frequency of birdsong unless I have my hearing aids in, their calls too shrill and high-pitched for my unaided ear.

In 2021 I moved with Tabitha to Oklahoma City; she got a job at Oklahoma Contemporary, one of the biggest art galleries in the state, as an art conservator. A library close to our house was the Ralph Ellison Library, which I discovered was named in honor of Ellison as it was his birth town.

In 1962, Ralph Ellison wrote an essay titled "On Bird, Bird-Watching and Jazz," exploring the life and music of his favorite jazz musician, Charlie Parker (who was nicknamed Bird).

The lack of specificity intrigued Ellison: Exactly what kind of bird is Charlie Parker? Ellison leans on his knowledge of bird sound and song, ruminating on the yardbird (chicken), mockingbird, and robin. How many of these sounds did Ellison first hear in Oklahoma? How subconsciously did Charlie Parker's sound root Ellison back in the land of his birth?

Oklahoma is vast, a striking landscape of lakes, grasslands, valleys, creeks, and dramatic skies. I had seen two snowstorms and an ice tornado within my first few months there, an equally terrifying and beautiful experience. Both storms left the park by our house eerily silent and iced over. The trees were so embedded in icicles they snapped in half; a patch of bright yellow flowers that had recently bloomed were iced in the frozen air, leaving the bright fire petals in tubes of ice. The weather in Oklahoma knew how to stage drama, all of it fleeting, rain or shine, storm or tornado. One taxi driver put it well: "If you don't like the weather in Oklahoma, just wait a minute." Nothing is fixed, every season passes through rapidly, sometimes all of them inside one hour. So it was in the aftermath of these dramatic weather events that I was tuned in to something new. I would see the birds returning on the walks I would take in the park as the ice melted. It would go from near-silence to gradual life as the birds and their families returned to their trees and their songs. In London when I went for walks, I turned my hearing aids off; in Oklahoma I started turning them up. The songs, their range of sound, would feed me something—some of the melodies were erratic and broken in intensity but I felt a slight bounce, a nourishing levity in what I would have once thought of as an overwhelm of sound; but these sounds in this context were almost ecstatic, the songs of birds that had survived and returned dizzy and chanting euphoric praise, sharing a lightness, the way the curve in the story of our lives can bend without breaking. This is nature's show. We are mere spectators.

I write down the names given to me, the names I've given myself, and all the unhealed hurts that I have been labeled with. I write "dumb," "stupid," "idiot," "not real deaf," "ugly." I write "baby signer" and "bush boy." I write "shame" again and again; I sign it—closed fist toward the face and then open the palm. I write "disappointment" and "I wish I could hear." I write "limited," "self-sufficient," all the labels that got stuck in my head with a punishing repetition. I write phrases I wish to turn down, erase forever, flat phrases that have no service for who or what I am: "hearing loss," "hearing impaired," I write "limited" again—words with fingers that point in one direction, at me. I think of David Wright exorcizing himself, renaming himself, of Goya consuming himself, and I burn each label, word, phrase, and watch it shrivel and disappear into smoke and fire. I write the word "forgive." I don't burn it; instead, I place it on the frame of the mirror on my bedroom wall. I sign it. Forgive: right index finger to mouth, then bring down right hand to left palm, both hands meet in a circular motion, as if something just said or thought is rubbed or washed away.

"Forgive me / my deafness for my own sound, how I mistook it for a wound / you could heal" is a line from Deaf poet Meg Day's lyrical and intimate poem "Elegy in Translation."

I resonate with this idea of having your own sound. I have been in many rooms when someone asks, "Can you hear that?" and I've heard nothing. I was in those English classes being taught how to write iambic pentameter, taught it as if it is the sole measure of sound and poetic value. I almost wept when I read Kamau Brathwaite for the first time and came across the line "the hurricane does not roar in pentameters." I resonated with that line so fiercely I slammed my fist on the table in the study area of the Poetry Library, immediately being shushed by the librarian. There are many layers to one's own sound. We all experience sound in a different way and often tuning in to our inner music can serve us more powerfully than the pathologies outside us. Our own sound hints at a need to nurture a kind of personal music in the noisy world of language.

Speaking of music, a memorable line of Day's poem goes, "So what / if Johnny Nash *can see clearly now Lorraine is gone*— I only wanted / to hear the sea." Mishearings are an obvious staple of deaf poetics, a way to honor one's own sound. "Lorraine" is a corruption of "the rain" from the song "I Can See Clearly Now." Even knowing that Meg Day is an American poet and happens to be listening to Johnny Nash's version of the song tells us something significant (I'm more familiar with Jimmy Cliff's cover of "I Can See Clearly Now"). Engaging with the physicality of sign language, an idea of "translation" comes into the poem. "My hands are bloated / with the name signs of my kin . . ." In the Deaf world, friends have sign names that can only be assigned to you by someone else in the Deaf community. Despite this specificity it's not something that alienates anyone because the verb "bloated" is active enough in multiple ways with "name signs"; it works as both a concrete and an abstract noun. These kinds of linguistic gymnastics are woven throughout the poem, using slant and internal rhymes and alliteration—techniques hard to pull off meaningfully—and contrast with the image near the beginning, the "fluke of their tongues." The poetic accomplishment here is far from a fluke; it's an intentional affirmation of one's own sound, a tongue-in-cheek lament, skilled and measured, written by a Deaf poet.

Deaf writing is not "woke," it's nothing new; deaf authors have been penning in print since Pierre Desloges in the 1700s and John Kitto in the 1800s. I wouldn't find these names in my formal education in my teens, I would find them while rummaging the shelves in the London Library in my late twenties.

What I have needed is a path, a link, a passage, maybe an ark, something that carries these names and lives to and through me in the present day so I know I exist, in the past, present, and into the future.

I'm not just writing about self-salvation but about the integration of deaf people, out of the margins and into mainstream society. In the UK, research from the National Deaf Children's Society reported that there are more deaf children in school now (in 2023) than when I left school in 2003, and yet, there are fewer deaf schools and support systems for them. It makes no sense.

I feel I was lucky to go to school when I did, it was almost a golden era for special educational needs (SEN) and deaf education in the UK, and yet, growing up, especially as a teenager, anxiety, shame, guilt encompassed large parts of my internal vocabulary. The way I spoke to myself inside my own head was loud and punishing:

I wish I could hear I wish I could hear I wish . . .

These exorcisms, these naming ceremonies, these poetic pursuits, these Deaf poets, all provide new language, balms for my old, heavy, unforgiving voice, countering some of my own ableist self-talk, nudging me out of judgment, toward a curiosity, an investigation about myself and a world of sound and silence filled with a life of poetic potential.

I sometimes imagine an all-hearing God, a white cloud with one tiny ear and one giant ear, neither needing help from hearing aids, neither missing any sound, and this all-hearing God heard enough of the world and decided to destroy the all-hearing world in a great flood, and we mere mortals needed passage to the Deaf world, to integrate it into a world we must share, a world where what is learned from speech and sign language and lip-reading and captioned screens in train stations and airports and hospital wards and classrooms is all part of the air, and my grandfather returned to Earth as a voice to sermonize our salvation. "Granddad J.K.," I'd say, "we need an ark to connect us to the D/deaf world, we need deliverance from the wrath of this all-hearing God," and Grandfather J.K. would ask, calmly, thoughtfully, as I feel the electric in my hearing aids meet the electricity of the question, "Who is on the ark?" And I'd say, "Granville Redmond is on the ark, his canvas wet with passing storms and luminous lakes; Dorothy Miles is on the ark, signing, speaking, writing all her gestures on deck; Johnnie Ray is on the ark and all his dancing static; David Wright, with or without deaf shame, is on the ark and so is Goya and all the animals in his 'Black Paintings'; owls, elephants, bats, dogs, bulls, and large cats, and all the clean and unclean beasts are on the ark; my mother's telephone is on the ark and so are all the teachers and interpreters of the deaf: Thomas Braidwood, Penny Wiles,

Renata, Deborah, Alfred Evelyn Clarke, Hashem Ghazal, Claudia Gordon, Antoinette Aiken, Tashi Widmer; forgers of good relationships, good listeners are on the ark!"

Grandfather J.K. would touch his mustache, knowing whom we were about to summon.

"Grandmother Barbara is on the ark, hands clasped, leaning back in her floral armchair, and so is Grandmother Darcas, literate in land, wood, and water; Donald Winnicott is on the ark and so is the kind patience of Mr. Barry and Mark the swimming coach with his gestured poolside instructions. Who else is on the ark? Thomas Gray's poems and my father's handmade sound systems; every smooth and distorted syllable from Blake to Brathwaite; every school of Miss Lou; every dub of Linton Kwesi Johnson and Jean 'Binta' Breeze, John Agard and Adrian Mitchell, Gil Scott-Heron, Mutabaruka, Michael Rosen; every talking drum blares like Beethoven on the ark; Zephaniah's megaphoned people power is on the ark; Malika's Poetry Kitchen and all her silver and yellow carnival colors are on the ark. Poetry Library librarians are on the ark whispering 'break a line' over all the scribbling poets' shoulders; Meg Day is on the ark and so is their phrase 'deaf kin,' Paddy Ladd's phrase 'Deafhood,' John Lee Clark's phrase 'hearing canon'; Aaron Williamson's phrase 'Deaf gain,' Harriet McBryde Johnson in her wheelchair is on the ark speaking and speaking and speaking, and John Kitto and Pierre Desloges and Jack Clemo's earthy hands are on the ark and, look, my old sign name 'R' Cap is on the ark and so is my new sign name—the BSL letter R that raises over the head to open all fingers out in the BSL word for *light, shower, sunrays*—all of it on the ark smelling like sweat, salt, rivers, oceans, blood and blood."

My son is two. He is outdoorsy, observant, wide-eyed, and when I walk him across the fields and parks near our rented house, he points excitedly and smiles when birds fly overhead. He's started noticing trees, pointing at their stance, the way some seem to hold themselves up in surrender, others seem frozen in dance, some seem withered, given up; my son observes the personality of nature, is alive to its expressions. As I pass the shaded trees with my son, I'm thinking of where I am, alive and hoping to offer him a wider, worldly education, one that speaks to and with his nature, something that makes us like the trees that surround us now as we walk through the fields of Hertfordshire, ten miles from Hemel Hempstead where my grandfather used to preach, writing his own poems on the back of his sermons, and I can't distinguish the bramble from the hawthorn but I know the silver birches (Birch, my father's family name) and I make a point to tap their trunks with my ring finger the way my father tapped lampposts when he walked past them, a sound, a gesture, something that seemed to make my father bounce, lighten his step.

All this is to say that I recognize the birch and the oak and I say *Birch* and *Oak* and it's October so I say *Autumn* because of the fallen burnt-orange leaves and the hard sundried mud and the brown wooden fence that I have pushed open to enter onto the particular field I come to on days like this, where darker green grass grows beside a path of lighter yellowy *Wizard of Oz*–like grass that shines in the high afternoon sun like a path leading us toward some majestic and unsayable thing, but my son, whose language is beginning, chants the only words he makes,

Ma-ma, Da-da, and his own name *I-ra, I-ra,* and as we reach the bench I unstrap him from the sling and put him on the ground and watch him reach toward the seat. I pick him up, place him on my lap, and do the only thing there is to do: face the path we've walked, notice the clouds sliding across the sky above the fields, and I point *hawk, crow, pigeon, swallow,* sounding out what I can in the country that appears before us.

ACKNOWLEDGMENTS

This book would not be possible without exchanges with other writers, poets, artists, activists, teachers, scholars, readers, and fellow investigators of missing sound in the D/deaf world, including Kevin Buckle, Grace Buckle, Jacqi Beckford, Ian Dhanoolal, Dr. Benjamin Braithwaite, Dr. Paddy Ladd, Sophie Stone, Sophie Woolley, Nadia Nadarajah, Toni Aiken, Lisa Kelly, Caro Parker, Paula Garfield, Rubbena Aurangzeb-Tariq, Omeima Mudawi-Rowlings, Ted Evans, Chris Fonseca, Signkid, Harry Jardine, Meg Day, Ilya Kaminsky, Saleem Hue Penny, John Lee Clark, Rose Ayling-Ellis, Sarah Katz, Louise Stern, Christopher Jon Heuer, Kate Rowley, christine sun kim, Daniel Jillings, Ann Jillings, Brian Duffy, Lily Bertrand-Webb, Pettra St. Hillaire, Dame Evelyn Glennie, Polly Dunbar, Joyce Dunbar, Liam O'Dell, Reece Cattermole, Shula Berrington, Rachael Boast, Dr. Kelly Fagan Robinson, Karl Knights, Zoë McWhinney, Charmaine Wombwell, Naomi Bottrill, Rezene Woldeyesus, Hermon Berhane, Herooda Berhane, Saffiatu Kamara, Emma Ripard, Nicole Bartolo, Douglas Ridloff, Lauren Ridloff, Jeffrey Mansfield, and Charlie Swinbourne.

You don't forget the teachers that care: Renata, Mr. Barry,

Dorothy Miles, Miss Walker, Miss Willis, Mr. Ferguson, Miss Mukassa, and all my teachers of the deaf and SEN units and the incredible NHS support I got from speech therapists and audiologists at the Donald Winnicott Centre and the Royal National Throat, Nose and Ear Hospital in the early 2000s, thank you. I give thanks to my mother, Rosemary Antrobus, and Hackney teacher of the deaf Penny Wiles, for the seeds they planted in my education.

To Malika Booker, Deanna Rodger, Gee, Simon Mole, Adam Kammerling, Jacob Sam-La Rose, Roger Robinson, Nick Makoha, Joelle Taylor, Hannah Lowe, Nathalie Teitler, Karen McCarthy-Woolf, Benjamin Zephaniah (we miss you), Gboyega Odujano (we miss you), Sharmilla Beezmohun, Linton Kwesi Johnson, Bernadine Evaristo, Margaret Busby, Anthony Joseph, Peter Kahn, Pádraig Ó'Tuama, Michael Rosen, and Jack Underwood—writing this book made me realize how much you changed my life in poetry, thank you.

Gratitude to Colin Grant and Kate Clanchy, who offered sound advice and encouragement on an early version of this manuscript. Special thanks to David Evans for helping find this book a home and to my agent, Niki Chang, who held me accountable to finishing this book.

Thanks to the editors at Granta for publishing a section of "Johnnie Ray" and to the commissioners at BBC Radio 3's *The Essay, Into the Wild* series, for including a section of "Sounding Out."

To my editors, Alexa von Hirschberg and Parisa Ebrahimi, for your care and belief, thank you.

To my co-parent, Tabitha Austin, who put in extra hours of childcare (visible and invisible labor) for our family while I wrote and traveled, thank you. This was not possible without you.

Ira, Daddy loves you.

Finally, readers, investigators, good luck finding your missing sounds.

R✹

NOTES

ix *Half-heard and half-created:* The William Wordsworth epigraph is lifted from "Fragment: Yet once again" but appears in a different form in the poem "Lines Composed a Few Miles above Tintern Abbey, on Revisiting the Banks of the Wye during a Tour. July 13, 1798."

xi *We have more senses:* The quote is mine and is lifted from "Deaf Poetics: A Conversation with Raymond Antrobus & Ilya Kaminsky," published in 2017 by Poetry International.

CHAPTER 1: THE FREQUENCIES ARE YOURS

13 *said his friend Charlie Chaplin:* Quote sourced from Scott A. Shields, PhD, and Mildred Albronda's curator talk at the Laguna Art Museum: www.youtube.com/watch?v=DXF1FhGL0MM.

CHAPTER 2: LIVIN' IN HACKNEY, NO ONE CAN JACK ME . . .

25 *the English performance artist and clown Jules Baker:* Some of the work created by Jules Baker and my mother, Rosie Antrobus, is mentioned in the book *Art Sex Music* by Cosey Fanni Tutti (Faber & Faber 2017).

30 *let's call him Calvin:* I was unable to confirm this story beyond anecdotes that I remember from my Aunt Avis and my dad, so I have told it as I remember it. I can't say for certain if a child with so-called delayed development would be in a Jamaican class for academically gifted students.

CHAPTER 4: THE QUIET EAR

64 *disabled not desirable:* This quote, taken from my journal as a teenager, is an example of ableist self-harm. Today, my D/deaf identity is claimed as a disabled identity too.

CHAPTER 5: CHOOSING MY LANE

84 *ponders Young:* It is important to clarify that there is *not* bountiful funding for Paralympic athletes, and many disabled athletes relate to the struggles that Young, as a Deaf athlete, is expressing. The overall system is making D/deaf and disabled people fight over scraps. Young makes very valid points about the divisions between different groups of athletes and the consequences for those that fall out of those categories, but it doesn't seem that the model of the "Deaflympics" remedies that; instead, it just provides a different version of a flawed and problematic system. John Loeppky wrote an excellent article on the Disability Debrief website entitled "Paralympic Paradoxes," which gives a more complex view on these dilemmas: www.disabilitydebrief.org/debrief/paralympic-paradoxes.

84 *Deaf swimmers like Young are in different lanes and races:* It is important to clarify that, yes, Deaf swimmers are disabled swimmers, but the categorizing of the different sporting organizations (Deaflympics, Paralympics, Olympics, etc.) confuses these distinctions. Swimmers with disabilities may find themselves racing able-bodied athletes on their way to qualifying for major tournaments.

CHAPTER 12: SOUNDING OUT

179 *fewer deaf schools and support systems for them:* This refers to infrastructural support for deaf, hard of hearing, and disabled peoples, including grants to hire BSL interpreters and access to adequate hearing technology, BSL lessons, and teachers of the deaf. It is important to stress that technically there is a distinction between wider accessibility and specific reasonable accommodations (adjustments made for individuals, based on individual needs).

179 *It makes no sense:* Unfortunately, it does make sense, just not a good kind of sense. Social inclusion is undermined by austerity measures that have gutted public services and individual disability benefits and allowances. The impact of this includes closing deaf schools and SEN departments and limiting the quality of support for deaf and hard of hearing students in mainstream schools. This is complicated by the fact that many deaf, hard of hearing, and disabled people prefer (often dogmatically) mainstream education, and there is some controversy over this (including pushback by deaf people).

ABOUT THE AUTHOR

RAYMOND ANTROBUS is the author of three poetry collections: *The Perseverance, All the Names Given,* and *Signs, Music.* Antrobus's poems have been added to GCSE syllabi, and his poetry has won the Ted Hughes Award, the Somerset Maugham Award, and *The Sunday Times* Young Writer of the Year Award. In 2019 he became the first ever poet to be awarded the Rathbone Folio Prize for best work of literature in any genre. He is also the author of two children's picture books, including *Can Bears Ski?,* which became the first story to be broadcast on the BBC entirely in British Sign Language.

Antrobus is an advocate for several D/deaf charities, including DeafKidz International and the National Deaf Children's Society.

Antrobus was elected a Fellow of the Royal Society of Literature in 2020 and appointed a Member of the Order of the British Empire in 2021.

Raymondantrobus.com

Instagram: @raymond_antrobus